Praise for Christy Harrison's
ANTI-DIET

"Nutritionist Christy Harrison, host of the podcast *Food Psych,* debuts with this impassioned and articulate plea for readers to reject 'diet culture' and reclaim their lives...Harrison's enlightening, heretical tract provides a new perspective on the dieting narrative that many take as gospel truth." —*Publishers Weekly*

"*Anti-Diet* is the 'diet' book you need to read...If you've been gearing up to embark on yet another diet, protocol, reset, or reboot come January 1, I have a different suggestion: Hit the pause button on that plan and read Christy Harrison's book. Harrison, a registered dietitian and journalist, thoroughly and elegantly lays out the strange origins of modern diet culture... then presents a path to truly holistic health that's based on self-care, not self-control." —Carrie Dennett, *Seattle Times*

"Brilliant! *Anti-Diet* should be required reading for every health professional and in every health-related class. Harrison bridges the gap between intuitive eating and social justice issues in an engaging and compassionate way. She exposes toxic diet culture—its evolution, who profits by it, and how it hurts you. Written with a friendly touch of sass, *Anti-Diet* is richly sourced with studies, stats, and interviews with experts. I highly recommend this book to help you dismantle diet culture and to heal your own relationship with food, mind, and body." —Evelyn Tribole, coauthor of *Intuitive Eating*

"A huge burden has been lifted: I no longer have to revise my first book to reflect current understanding! Christy Harrison beat me to it. I'm blown away by how good *Anti-Diet* is. Through a social-justice lens, well-researched and smart science, captivating storytelling, and practical advice, this book will help you reclaim your life from the throttle of diet culture."

—Lindo Bacon, author of *Health at Every Size*
and coauthor of *Body Respect*

"As compassionate as it is scholarly, *Anti-Diet* goes deep to expose the sordid underbelly of the diet culture, but it doesn't leave you there. With healing-oriented strategies that address your physical, emotional, and social self, this book will leave you armed with ways to reclaim all that dieting has taken from you, and give you a new perspective that is empowering and sustainable."

—Jenna Hollenstein, MS, RDN, CDN,
author of *Eat to Love*

"*Victory!* Christy Harrison epically takes down diet culture and explains why the cards are stacked against all of us who still believe a smaller body is the only way to improve health and create a better life. Diet culture sucks, but you can take meaningful action: Read this book. Stop dieting. Start being good to yourself."

—Rebecca Scritchfield, RDN, author of *Body Kindness*

"If you've ever wondered how we landed in this current wellness-obsessed, sugar-and-gluten-fearing moment of entrenched food anxiety, *Anti-Diet* is a must-read. Harrison traces the history of modern diet culture, busts deeply rooted myths, and exposes the inherent biases of modern weight research. She also offers clear, practical advice for all of us trying to disentangle ourselves from diets and make peace with food."

—Virginia Sole-Smith, author of *The Eating Instinct*

"This book will forever change the way you see the world and live your life. Thank God for Christy Harrison."

—Jes Baker, author of *Things No One Will Tell Fat Girls*

"Most diet and wellness books claim to address mind, body, and spirit, but in fact they are just about body. Thank goodness for Christy Harrison, whose empathetic book reveals oppressive diet culture for what it truly is and offers a genuinely holistic alternative."
—Alan Levinovitz, author of *The Gluten Lie*

"Please read this book! *Anti-Diet* is the book to end all diet books and will be a game changer for so many people. Harrison is an expert on this subject and leaves no stone unturned in exposing how insidious and harmful diet culture is—and in teaching readers how to opt out of the madness."
—Caroline Dooner, author of *The F*ck It Diet*

ANTI-DIET

RECLAIM YOUR TIME, MONEY, WELL-BEING, AND HAPPINESS THROUGH INTUITIVE EATING

CHRISTY HARRISON, MPH, RD

Little, Brown Spark
New York Boston London

For Mom and Dad, who gave me life, language, and
a penchant for challenging authority

———————————————————

Little, Brown Spark
Hachette Book Group
1290 Avenue of the Americas, New York, NY 10104
littlebrownspark.com

Originally published in hardcover by Little, Brown Spark, December 2019
First Little, Brown Spark paperback edition, December 2021

Little, Brown Spark is an imprint of Little, Brown and Company, a division of
Hachette Book Group, Inc. The Little, Brown Spark name and logo are
trademarks of Hachette Book Group, Inc.

The publisher is not responsible for websites (or their content) that are not
owned by the publisher.

The Hachette Speakers Bureau provides a wide range of authors for
speaking events. To find out more, go to hachettespeakersbureau.com or call
(866) 376-6591.

ISBN 9780316420358 (hc) / 9780316420372 (pb)
LCCN 2019940323

Printing 1, 2021

LSC-C

Printed in the United States of America

Contents

ANTI-DIET

Introduction

Like the vast majority of American women, I've had a rocky relationship with food at various points in my life. I somehow made it through childhood and adolescence without any eating issues, despite having had the usual body-image insecurities that come with growing up female (and increasingly growing up any gender) in our society. I was raised in the San Francisco Bay Area in the 1980s and '90s, and my parents and most of their friends were middle-class recovering hippies who eschewed many of the '50s-era social conventions and gender roles they'd been brought up with. Yet pretty much all the adult women in my life were dieting or "watching what they ate," just like their mothers before them. As the girls my age began to hit puberty, they started dieting, too. But not me. Although I was insecure about my changing body, I wasn't what society considered fat, or even chubby. I never had a parent or doctor tell me to lose weight, and wasn't bullied for my size or shape. Those were unearned privileges I didn't even know I had until much later—privileges that unfortunately weren't afforded to some of my friends. A few fell prey to eating disorders and went to treatment, while others muddled along on their own.

In high school I started hanging out with the "alternative" kids, the ones who listened to punk rock and ska on seven-inch records and had lots of piercings. I got some piercings and a record player, too, and emblazoned the cover with punk stickers—including one that said, "You CAN be too rich and too thin" with a drawing of a skeletal stick figure trying in vain to lift a huge bag of money. That whole time I was pretty oblivious to the disordered eating going on around me—partly because I was going through my own struggles with family dysfunction, social anxiety, and general teenage rebellion, but also because I was still insulated by the privilege of living in a relatively thin body. Years later I came to learn that a number of my punk-rock friends had been dieting and struggling with eating disorders. While my sister and I would sometimes call each other *fat* as an insult, I didn't take those comments seriously, and it never even occurred to me to try to lose weight—although the concept of weight loss was all around me. I had a massive appetite, and it became a point of pride rather than a source of shame simply because of my size. "You can eat whatever you want," my friends would groan as I plowed through boxes of cereal, cartons of ice cream, and even tubes of cake frosting as after-school snacks. My best friend's mother joked that I was a human garbage disposal because I'd gladly polish off anything she deemed too "fattening" to keep in the house.

In my early twenties, that state of general body-size acceptance came to an end. I was at UC Berkeley for college—not nearly far enough away from home to satisfy my wanderlust—and so I signed up to do a study-abroad program in Paris for my junior year. While I was there, I started on a new birth-control pill and gained a little bit of weight, and suddenly everything I'd been told my whole life about food and size came bubbling to the surface. It didn't matter that I was still objectively small, with all the freedoms that Western culture affords people in smaller bodies (such as being able to fit easily into an airplane or theater seat, buy clothes in mainstream stores, and walk down the street without having insults hurled at me for daring to leave the house). I did exactly what most people do when they grow up in a society obsessed with weight loss and then find themselves unable to button their pants: I went on a diet.

Dieting felt like unlocking a new level in life. I started getting compliments on my weight loss left and right, both in Paris and when I returned home to Berkeley in the summer of 2002. By that point the United States had entered the Age of Atkins, and suddenly I was bonding with friends and family over low-carb recipes and calorie counting. A missing piece of my social life finally seemed to fall into place: now I had a way to connect with strangers at the store, acquaintances at parties, and colleagues on my college-magazine staff. I'd always felt awkward around people I didn't know well, especially in groups, but dieting gave me a way in — it was the bridge between small talk and intimacy that I never knew I needed. People wanted to know my weight-loss secrets, and I was happy to blab them all over town.

The dream didn't last long, though. Within a couple of months, my shiny new life folded in on itself. I began sneaking into the kitchen most nights for binges on "forbidden" food — which was pretty much just my roommate's food, since I'd gotten rid of all the other carbs in the house. The guilt I felt for stealing from her was no match for my appetite, which was like a monster I was powerless to control. The next day I'd double down on the diet and exercise to compensate. Wash, rinse, repeat. I felt like shit, mentally and physically, and I knew the binges were disordered — but when I went to see a therapist about them, she just told me everyone has some eating issues and I was being too hard on myself. I also lost my period for more than a year, which I now know was my body's natural response to restrictive eating, but at the time I couldn't see it. I looked for something, *anything*, that could account for my hormones being so out of whack: Was it my thyroid? Was it gluten? And I searched for what I assumed were the deep emotional reasons why I lost control around bread. What was *wrong* with me that I couldn't just eat normally?

Nothing, it turns out. My body was functioning exactly the way bodies are designed to function on a diet: they do everything in their power to restore the lost weight and reverse what they perceive as famine. Today, as a dietitian specializing in disordered eating, I've seen the substantial scientific evidence that intentional weight loss almost never lasts and that it harms both physical and mental health.[1] Dieting—the act of changing your eating and exercise habits in order to lose weight and ostensibly improve your health—is a lot more likely to end in a host of problems (including rebound bingeing, food obsession, and weight regain, as it did for me) than it is to result in a slimmer, "better" you.[2] Not just *re*gain, actually; as many as two-thirds of people who embark on weight-loss efforts end up gaining more weight than they lost.[3] In the long run, intentional weight loss takes most people in the opposite direction they thought they were going.

Despite the strong evidence against dieting—which has been covered over the years in hundreds of books, articles, talk shows, and other media outlets—millions of people still do it. The research firm Marketdata reported in early 2019 that the diet industry was worth more than $72 billion, a record high.[4] In recent years 68 percent of Americans have dieted for some length of time, mostly making up their own weight-loss plans or "lifestyle changes" rather than following formal diets to the letter, according to 2016 data by global research firm The NPD Group. A close cousin of dieting is disordered eating: using behaviors such as fasting, chronic restrained eating, restricting major food groups, vomiting, or laxatives to try to lose weight, and/or bingeing, as many people do as a result of dieting, all without engaging in any of those behaviors frequently or consistently enough to meet the criteria for a full-blown eating disorder. A 2008 survey by researchers at the University of North Carolina at Chapel Hill in conjunction with *Self* magazine found that 65 percent of American women between the ages of 25 and 45 have some form of disordered eating, and that another 10 percent would meet the criteria for eating disorders (although far fewer are actually diagnosed). Clinicians specializing in eating and body image report that these issues are on the rise in men as well, and transgender people are actually more likely than cisgender folks to have both diagnosed eating disorders and disordered-eating behaviors.[5] In short, people of all stripes are feeling pressure to change their body size by any means necessary.

Why are we so wedded to dieting when it so clearly doesn't work—and is even hurting us? Shouldn't we know better by now? In my work I've come to see that it's not just an issue of knowledge, although that's a part of it. It's also an issue of culture. Specifically, *diet culture*—a system of beliefs that equates thinness, muscularity, and particular body shapes with health and moral virtue; promotes weight loss and body reshaping as a means of attaining higher status; demonizes certain foods and food groups while elevating others; and oppresses people who don't match its supposed picture of "health."

By and large, Western culture is diet culture. This way of thinking about food and bodies is so embedded in the fabric of our society, in so many different forms, that it can be hard to recognize. It masquerades as health, wellness, and fitness. It cloaks itself as connection. Diet culture is what I'd stumbled into when I started bonding with people over restrictive ways of eating. Diet culture is what caused my friends to compliment my weight loss, and what kept me coming back for more even when it was clearly harming my well-being. Diet culture is what makes some of my clients skip birthday parties out of fear that they'll have to eat cake. It's what made some of their parents put them on diets before they were old enough to remember their birthday parties.

Diet culture is consuming us. In the thousands of conversations I've had with people about their relationships with food and their bodies, I've seen the same themes emerge again and again: People have lost years of their lives to dieting and disordered eating. They've spent thousands and even hundreds of thousands of dollars on diet products and programs that didn't work and just left them more hopeless. They've tried to lose weight or change their eating because health professionals or magazine articles told them to, only to end up sicker than they started out—and usually heavier, too (although weight isn't an indicator of health, as we'll discuss in Chapter 5). They haven't really *been there* at weddings, funerals, graduations, honeymoons, and countless other important moments because thoughts of food and weight were consuming their minds.

Diet culture stole their lives.

It has stolen millions of lives, and it stole mine for more than a decade, too. My disordered eating continued after I graduated from college; it followed me into my career as a journalist. In my first full-time job at an eco-lifestyle magazine in New York City, I had trouble concentrating on the articles I was supposed to be writing and editing because I couldn't stop thinking about food. I was also eating so little during the day that my brain was starved of the energy it needed to function. I spent all my time outside work researching restaurants, going on "food adventures" with my then-boyfriend, and having epic binges that inadvertently gave my body all the food it was missing—and then overexercising to "make up" for what I perceived as my failure to "eat right."

Unable to stop myself from daydreaming about food or perseverating about nutrition at work, I decided to channel those interests into my writing. I started pitching more and more food- and nutrition-related stories at the magazine (ironically called *Plenty*), and after a couple of years I left to do freelance writing solely focused on food and nutrition—all while struggling with what felt like the shameful secret of my "out-of-control" eating. I became a food writer with an eating disorder. To be honest, I'm 99 percent sure I would have pursued an entirely different journalistic beat if my eating hadn't been so disordered. I had lots of other long-standing interests — politics, psychology, performing arts, social justice — and I'd never even cared that much about food until I started restricting it (which, at the time, I wouldn't or couldn't admit that I was doing).

Fortunately, working as a food writer did help me start to loosen up on those restrictions, especially when I got another full-time job as an editor at *Gourmet.* There I was surrounded mostly by people who had peaceful relationships with food, sometimes for two to three meals a day — our hours were long, and the editors often went out to eat together after work. I also never knew when I was going to be called down to the test kitchen to taste a recipe that would be running alongside one of my stories. I couldn't be weird about it; I *had* to eat. But I was by no means fully recovered, and I continued to feel extremely guilty about my eating and do low-level dieting behaviors to compensate for how I was eating at work.

Then, in 2009, amid rumblings that *Gourmet* was going to close (which it eventually did — RIP), I went back to school at New York University to study public-health nutrition and get my registered dietitian's license. That definitely exacerbated my food issues, at least at first. It felt like everyone around me was eating "perfectly," and to be a good student I had to as well — so I ramped up on the food rules, and my binges consequently became more frequent and intense. But then, in my second semester of grad school, I decided that in my copious spare time I was going to write a book about emotional eating. I never finished the book proposal, but in researching the topic I stumbled on *Intuitive Eating* by Evelyn Tribole and Elyse Resch, and that book both blew my mind and helped me reconnect with the easygoing relationship with food that I'd had while growing up. In my years of living in New York I'd also finally found a good therapist, and she helped me untangle my lingering food issues and the underlying beliefs that were driving them.

I was ultimately able to recover from diet culture by giving up all forms of dieting, consistently eating enough and not restricting any food groups, making peace with my body, and learning to approach food and exercise from a place of self-care rather than a place of self-control. In *Anti-Diet* I'll share how you can do the same—at any size. (It may take extra practice and support for people in larger bodies because of the weight stigma inherent in diet culture, but I promise it's possible, and in this book you'll hear from lots of folks who've been able to do it.) We'll discuss how diet culture—which I've nicknamed the Life Thief—has infiltrated the health-and-wellness field, and how to tell the difference between diet culture and self-care practices that truly support well-being. You'll learn why intentional weight loss is nearly impossible to sustain, and why letting go of efforts to shrink your body can improve your health, no matter your size. I'll show you how to tune in to your body's cues about how to eat, and tune out all the noise coming from diet culture. I'll share why you need to give a big middle finger to the Life Thief in order to reclaim your right to have *enough*—enough food to feel truly satisfied, and enough mental space to pursue the things that really matter in life. I'll also help you recognize that you *are* enough exactly as you are, and that you don't need to shrink your body or change your eating to be worthy. We'll look at why mental health is just as important as physical health, and how you can heal both your mind and your body from the destructive influences of the Life Thief.

A few things you won't find in this book: weights, measurements, calorie counts, or detailed descriptions of diet and exercise plans. These kinds of specifics have been shown to hinder people's ability to recover from disordered eating and diet culture; they only trigger harmful comparisons and provide a "how-to manual" of new disordered behaviors to try. Obviously, that's the opposite of what I want; *Anti-Diet* is meant to help you with your food issues, not make them worse. So just as I do in my podcast, *Food Psych,* I'll deliberately omit those problematic details here. (I can't guarantee the same for every study or article I reference, so if you decide to delve into the original sources that I cite in the endnotes, be forewarned that many of them contain triggering details—and proceed at your own risk.) If you're reading along and you find yourself really wanting to know, say, a person's exact weight or clothing size, recognize that this desire is actually a product of diet culture—and that's what I'm going to help you move away from in this book. As you'll discover in Chapter 1, there was a time not long ago when people didn't have access to information about weight, calories, or clothing sizes; in my view society would hugely benefit if we could stop having those details be a part of everyday life.

You'll also see some language that's unusual for a book of this kind. I'm not talking just about the swearing: I use the words *overweight* and *obese* only within quotation marks, because those terms—as well as the concept of an "obesity epidemic"—have a troubling history, which I'll discuss in Chapter 1. These words stigmatize people in larger bodies and treat body size like a disease, which is apt to be more harmful to people's health than weight itself (as I'll make clear throughout the book, with an in-depth discussion in Chapter 5). Instead, I typically use the phrase *people in larger bodies* or *higher-weight people* to emphasize the fact that body size is a neutral trait, the way we say *people with brown hair* or *taller people,* and to highlight the fact that we're all just temporary inhabitants of these bodies that we use to move through the world.

You'll also hear from a number of people who embrace the word *fat* as a neutral descriptor for their size, and—in the spirit of the fat-acceptance movement—you'll see me use that term when my sources self-identify that way. I don't generally use *fat* as a descriptor outside that context, only because I recognize the traumatic memories it can stir up to hear a smaller-bodied person labeling others with a word that may have been cast your way as an epithet in the past. Still, I truly believe the word should carry no stigma, and that diet culture is the only reason it does. In Chapter 1 you'll learn how fatness once had positive connotations, and why that changed over time. You'll also learn a bit about the birth and history of the movement to reclaim *fat* as an identity rather than an insult.

Speaking of language, I strive to use terminology that's as gender-inclusive as possible, because the reality is that people of *all* genders struggle under the pressures of diet culture. Cisgender women, trans folks, and gender-nonconforming people generally bear the brunt of those pressures, but plenty of cisgender men grapple with food and body issues as well. Scientific and historical studies typically still divide participants into binary gender categories, though, so when discussing science and history I'll adopt whatever terms are reported in the research (typically just "women" and "men"). And of course when quoting sources I'll let their words stand.

Some of what you'll read here may challenge deeply held beliefs, and some of it will likely feel like a huge relief. For anyone who's been on the yo-yo diet cycle, this book will likely provide a renewed sense of freedom and possibility that there is another way to live, but it may also bring up some sadness as you recall the traumatic experiences you've had with diet culture. For those who've never lived in larger bodies, as well as that small percentage of people who've been weight-loss "success stories," this book might evoke some uncomfortable feelings about how you may have participated in diet culture or perpetuated weight stigma. It may also elicit some resistance and defensiveness, especially when I call out particular diets or "lifestyle changes" by name or discuss the ways in which diet culture masquerades as health and wellness. If any of that discomfort or resistance comes up for you, I hope you're able to sit with it and keep reading, allowing yourself to be open to a different point of view that could change your life for the better.

For everyone, my wish is that this book will help you understand your own struggles with food and dieting as part of a larger cultural context, recognize the many faces of diet culture, and develop the tools to take back your life once and for all.

PART I

The Life Thief

CHAPTER 1

The Roots of Diet Culture

Diet culture is a slippery thing. Some would argue that it doesn't exist anymore—that today everyone *knows* diets don't work, and that the average citizen of twenty-first-century Western culture is more concerned with health and wellness than thinness. "It's not a diet, it's a healthy lifestyle," today's weight-loss ads intone. "I don't diet, I just eat *real* food," social media's self-styled nutrition gurus declare. The thing is, though modern-day diets may disavow the term, they're part of the same belief system that brought us SlimFast and SnackWell's, and that keeps us chasing after an elusive "ideal" body size and shape. They're still part of diet culture. And as with any cultural phenomenon, in order to truly understand it we have to understand its history. We can't recognize how contemporary diet culture is harming us—or learn how to heal from it—without going back to its roots. Not only is the story of diet culture's development fascinating, but it holds important keys to unlocking the Life Thief's hold on us today.

For most of human existence, no one dreamed of restricting their food intake to lose weight. Getting *enough* food was the main concern, and plumpness signified prosperity and well-being. Fat on the body meant higher social status, a better chance of weathering famine and disease, and a greater likelihood of fertility. Thinness meant poverty, illness, and death.

Two of the earliest known sculptures of human beings—the

Venus of Hohle Fels and the *Venus of Willendorf*—depict big, round, feminine bodies with huge breasts and rolls of fat on their bellies and sides. Numerous kings, pharaohs, gods, and goddesses in the ancient world were depicted with fat bodies, symbolizing their fertility, divinity, and prestige.[1] Though religions have long issued warnings about gluttony and engaged in ritual fasting and asceticism, these practices weren't about weight loss for its own sake or the effects of eating on a person's size, but about how bodily pleasure was thought to compromise the soul.[2] Fasting was penance—a way of making up for all the times you had screwed up that year, rather than a way of punishing your body for being too large. In fact, at one time in the early nineteenth century gluttony was widely believed to cause food malabsorption and weight *loss,* rather than weight gain. (This belief came about because European visitors to the U.S. observed that white Americans were thinner than their European counterparts, and that these Americans also ate more food, more quickly, and more often.)

Today, in some parts of the world—especially those that are relatively insulated from Western beauty ideals—fatness is still seen as desirable. Anthropologist Rebecca Popenoe, who has spent years doing fieldwork in the Sahara desert, explains that a fat body is the ultimate symbol of beauty, prosperity, and health for women in Niger and Mauritania, to the point where many mothers deliberately try to fatten their daughters—and sometimes even force-feed them. Fatness signifies beauty and health for indigenous groups in parts of South America as well. By one estimate, 81 percent of human societies in recorded history have had beauty ideals that favored larger-bodied women.[3] The data on beauty ideals for men is more scant, but among the dozen or so societies with available evidence, virtually all of them have a preference for large body size (usually also accompanied by muscularity) in men.[4]

In the grand scheme of things, then, demonizing fatness is

an anomaly, limited to a few historical periods. One such period is classical antiquity—Ancient Greece and Rome—when the seeds of modern-day diet culture were planted. In that time of relative prosperity, there was a lot of anxiety about what abundance meant. Moderation and balance in all things came to be seen as a virtue, and any level of excess was a flaw to be corrected. So when it came to eating, overindulgence was deemed a moral failing; food was to be consumed exclusively for fuel, not for pleasure, and fatness was viewed as a symbol of moral corruption.[5] The Latin word *obesus*—the root of the English *obesity*—was coined in that period, and translates as "having eaten until fat."

This cultural fatphobia also intertwined with thinking about health. The Ancient Greek physician Galen, for example, believed that fatness was a sign of a malformed spirit.[6] In the "four humors" theory of medicine that became popular in that era (which held that health was achieved by balancing four essential elements in the body: black bile, yellow bile, blood, and phlegm), fatness was seen as an imbalance that needed to be corrected through arcane eating and exercise practices. Hippocrates—generally considered the father of Western medicine, and the namesake of the Hippocratic oath—popularized this belief, as well as the idea that fatness was a disease.[7] But there are many contradictions in the Greco-Roman view of fat bodies: Hippocrates (or possibly one of his disciples) also wrote, "In all maladies, those who are fat about the belly do best."[8]

Speaking of contradictions, the ancients generally didn't find thinness aesthetically appealing, and had a preference for "fat in moderation"—a beauty standard that still excluded lots of people, but wasn't nearly as impossible to live up to as today's thin ideal. And a linguistic analysis of Greek and Latin terms for *fat* and *thin* reveals that *fat* was frequently synonymous with prosperity and fertility, whereas *thin* was generally used to signify poverty and weakness.[9] So the Greeks and Romans were clearly ambivalent about what fatness "meant." As much as they may have believed that being larger-bodied was both a moral failing and a health problem, they didn't demonize fatness across the board.

After the fall of Rome, the notion of body fat as a symptom to be cured went mostly underground for a long time. The seeds of diet culture lay dormant, and fatness generally returned to being considered a positive trait, or at least a morally neutral one. Although there are some examples of thinness being prized in certain circles in the Middle Ages, there was no unified, institutionalized stigma against larger bodies until much more recently.

Meanwhile, although food has probably never been freighted with as much moral baggage as it is today, there were several periods in history when ideas about "good" and "bad" (or "right" and "wrong") ways of eating emerged. One of those periods is, again, classical antiquity. Our word *diet* comes from the Ancient Greek *diaita,* a term that did not enter widespread use until Hippocrates and his fellow physicians started using it in medical texts, primarily to refer to eating, drinking, and exercise habits (and occasionally also to bathing and sexual practices).[10]

Diaita is often translated as "way of life," but those early medical writings reveal the common usage of the word corresponds more closely to "regimen"—a system of rules governing behavior. The way Ancient Greek doctors saw it, anyone who didn't follow those rules properly (including the special rules that were supposed to apply depending on a person's constitution, the time of year, and the person's health status) was intellectually and morally inferior. Consider this passage from Hippocrates: "Those who do not use medicine—barbarians and a small number of Greeks—maintain (when they are sick) the same diet as those in health, only following their pleasure, and would neither forgo nor restrict the satisfaction of any of their desires, or even reduce the quantity."[11] In other words, people who don't follow the "proper" diet—which includes reducing the amount they eat in response to illness, and reject-ing pleasure in favor of health—are basically uncivilized brutes.

In another passage by Hippocrates, he argues that at the start of human existence people ate essentially the same things as animals, and their health suffered for it—and then progress marched forward until, what do you know, it arrived at the apex of sophistication that was the regimen recommended by Ancient Greek doctors. The implication is clear: eating anything other than the correct *diaita* made people less than fully human. The term *diet*, then, was bound up from the start with ideas about morality, restriction, the renunciation of pleasure, and the supe-riority of certain races.

The other key period in Western history when moralistic ideas about food came into vogue was in the days of Christopher Columbus—early modern colonialism. For the colonizers, this was a time filled with anxieties about how to live in an unfamil-iar environment among unfamiliar people (although of course things were far worse for those being colonized). Columbus and his fellow conquistadors feared that coming into contact with these new lands and their occupants would cause settlers to get sick and die—perhaps a justified fear, given that so many of them did (as did the indigenous peoples). To ensure this didn't happen, the Spanish colonizers believed they needed to eat the "right" food—specifically European food, which they thought would protect them from the excessively damp conditions in the Americas.[12] (The "four humors" theory was still prevalent in medicine at the time, and climate supposedly affected health by altering the humoral balance.) Spanish settlers insisted that indigenous foods made them sick because of this imbalance. Never mind the fact that the settlers ate these foods at pretty much every meal without incident; whenever illness struck, they were quick to blame the food.

What's more, as the colonizers started to form ideas about

race based on their contact with new peoples, they also began to believe that food helped *create* the physical distinctions between Europeans and the "others" they were encountering. That is, the Spaniards thought their bodies looked different than indigenous people's bodies because they ate differently—an early colonial example of the belief that "you are what you eat"—and that if they started eating the "bad" local foods, their bodies would literally transform to look like the people they were colonizing. That seemed less than ideal to the Spaniards, who also believed they had been sent by God to "civilize" these distant lands, and that even their appearance was a mark of this chosen status.[13] So in order to maintain their perceived divine right to lord it over everyone else, the conquistadors believed they had to keep eating the "correct" foods.

Those early modern colonial ideas about "good" and "bad" food, along with ideas from classical antiquity about the "correct" way to eat and the "right" size to be, began to commingle and germinate in the fertile ground of the nineteenth-century United States, which is when diet culture as we know it was born.

Industrialization and Its Discontents

Between the late eighteenth and early twentieth centuries, the U.S. saw an explosion in production, manufacturing, and technology known as the American Industrial Revolution, which had profound effects on society and culture. The original Industrial Revolution started in Britain in the mid-1700s and made its way across the pond in 1789, when a British textile manufacturer used smuggled designs to build the first industrial cotton mill in the U.S.[14] From there, textile and clothing production became increasingly mechanized, and by the 1820s ready-made clothes in standardized sizes began to take over the market.[15] Until that point, nearly everyone had been wearing custom-made clothes—rich or poor, going to a seamstress or sewing your own clothes was the only option. With the industrialization of clothing production, though, clothes were no longer made to fit your body and your precise measurements; now you had to choose your size from a limited array of mass-produced designs and hope for the best. Cue body shame and comparisons with your friends.

Meanwhile, the idea that food could play a role in health started to become more mainstream, thanks to Presbyterian minister and popular speaker Sylvester Graham (namesake of the cracker). In the mid-1830s, Graham began to advocate abstinence from alcohol, caffeine, and even meat and condiments, claiming that these substances were bad for people's health. He argued that "overstimulation" was the quintessential illness of the industrial age, preaching that a diet of austere, bland, non-stimulating foods was the key to both health and moral virtue. In Graham's view, spices, meat, sugar, caffeine, alcohol, and even yeasted bread and condiments led not only to indigestion and illness, but also to sexual "excess" (including both masturbation and too much sex between married couples) and general civil unrest. "Gluttony, and not starvation, is the greatest of all causes of evil," he wrote in 1838. Graham's beliefs epitomized the early Protestant worldview that advocated the denial of pleasure, the importance of self-control, and the triumph of reason over emotion. Through that lens, enjoying food was seen as a dangerous form of decadence.

In an origin story that harks back to colonial ideas about "good" and "bad" foods and also sounds eerily similar to many "wellness" bloggers today, Graham claimed that eating the "wrong" foods had caused him all kinds of health problems earlier in life, and that he had healed himself by cutting out those foods. Never mind that he had endured the kind of childhood trauma that would cause *anyone's* health to suffer, no matter what they ate: By the time young Sylvester was eight years old, his father had died and his mother had been declared "deranged." Graham bounced around among his older siblings' homes and neighbors' farms for the rest of his childhood, becoming an angry, bitter, chronically exhausted young man.[16] As an adult, he built his diet around what he deemed to be the only wholesome options: bran bread, plain rice, tapioca, sago (a kind of pudding made from palm flour), sauceless vegetables, and a few fruits. It wasn't intended as a weight-loss diet—in fact, Graham thought it would create robust bodies as well as wholesome minds—but given its austerity, people at the time worried that it would cause its followers to waste away.[17] In response, Graham and his acolytes (called "Grahamites") began weighing themselves regularly to prove that the diet allowed them to maintain their weight.

The Grahamites' records show that they more or less achieved that goal over the long term, even if some initial weight loss occurred for certain people. (That's basically true of all diets, as we'll discuss in Chapter 3.) These writings not only helped Graham refute the charges of starving his followers, they also provide the first evidence of a group of Americans tracking their body weight.[18] This routine weighing was quite a feat, given that scales weren't very common at the time (more on that shortly).

Race, Class, and Body Size

Industrialization soon led to urbanization—people moving into cities to work in the factories and offices that kept popping up. From 1850 to 1900 the percentage of Americans living in cities more than doubled, and by 1920 more Americans would live in cities than in the countryside.[19] Millions of people were clamoring for work, including a huge new wave of immigrants in the mid- to late 1800s. Industrialization also led to increased food production, which meant that food became available to a greater number of people for less labor than ever before.[20]

Some people thought this was all admirable progress, but American culture as a whole was awash in anxiety about what these changes meant—particularly when it came to immigration. The emerging white middle class was looking for ways to assert and maintain a dominant position in relation to the new immigrants, and body size became a key point of comparison. "Part of the rise of a thinner ideal to define a middle-class American citizen was this contradistinction to the 'stout, sturdy' immigrants," says cultural historian Emily Contois, who studies the nexus between gender and diet culture in American history. In other words, the anxious middle class started thinking of thinness as a mark of social status.

The nineteenth century also saw emerging theories about race and evolution that categorized people into a racial hierarchy based on which groups were supposedly more "civilized" or "evolved." The scientists doing the categorizing were predominantly white men of Northern European descent (including, most famously, British naturalist Charles Darwin beginning in the 1830s), and guess which group they claimed was at the top of the hierarchy? As important as evolutionary theory was when it came to explaining how we all came to be on this planet, it was also used in overtly racist ways, to justify the white Anglo-European male domination of other cultures and genders that had been going on for centuries. Evolutionary theory became a "scientific" way of upholding the status quo. White, Northern European women were deemed to be a step down from men on the evolutionary ladder, followed by Southern Europeans (again with the women a step down from the men), then people of color from countries that early biologists and anthropologists considered "semi-civilized" or "barbaric," and finally, at the bottom, Native Americans and Africans, whom they considered "savages."[21]

As part of their process of creating this bogus evolutionary hierarchy, nineteenth-century scientists started cataloguing the physical traits and cultural norms they saw in different societies. They decided that fatness was a marker of "savagery" because it appeared more frequently in the people of color they observed, whereas thinness supposedly appeared more frequently in white people, men, and aristocrats. In particular, fatness was said to be linked to blackness—an idea that started to take hold of the popular imagination in both Europe and the U.S. in the nineteenth century.[22] Scientific writings from this period obsessively catalogued and measured the fatness of people from supposedly "primitive" societies, and of women in general. Women of all ethnicities were believed to be at greater "risk" of fatness, which was taken as further evidence of their supposed evolutionary inferiority. Thus, belief in a hierarchy of ethnic groups, with white men at the top, led to a growing demonization of fatness starting in the mid-1800s.

These racist beliefs influenced our gender norms as well, including the definitions of what it means to "look male," "look female," and "look androgynous." Because thinness was deemed "more evolved" (given its supposed association with masculinity and whiteness), men with lots of fat on their bodies began to be seen as both less masculine and less morally upstanding. And whereas fatness or curviness was seemingly associated with femininity, the idea that larger bodies were inferior eventually translated to the idea that even women shouldn't be "too" fat or curvy. As sociologist Sabrina Strings explains in her 2019 book, *Fearing the Black Body*, this prohibition on fatness was especially strong for white, middle-class Protestant women, who were instructed on "temperance" by dietary reformers such as Sylvester Graham, and told that "excessive" eating was both immoral and detrimental to their beauty, as it would lead to having a body more like those of African or Irish women.[23]

Today these racist beauty ideals still affect not only cisgender people but those elsewhere on the gender spectrum. As nonbinary trans psychologist and activist Sand Chang puts it, "The ideals that we have for what trans bodies are supposed to look like are based on white, skinny, model-looking people, and it really excludes folks who are fat, disabled, and people of color. There are so many ways in which these dominant norms and dominant representations of trans identity don't leave room for the vast majority of us"—including nonbinary people who don't quite match society's idea of what it means to "look" nonbinary.

These days, diet culture pushes the narrative that the reason we stigmatize larger bodies is because higher weight "causes" poor health. In reality, though, fat bodies were deemed "uncivilized" and therefore undesirable long before the medical and scientific communities began to label them a health risk around the turn of the twentieth century.[24] Fatphobic beliefs pre-dated health arguments. In fact, through the end of the nineteenth century (as for most of human history) doctors held that larger bodies were *healthier*. Anyone who wanted to pursue weight loss had to go up against the medical establishment.

Weighty Matters

One such person was William Banting, Britain's first weight-loss guru. In 1862 Banting had retired from a successful career as a funeral director for British royalty and seemed set for life, but he couldn't shake his frustration with his weight.[25] He went to a number of doctors about it, but like the vast majority of physicians in that era, they thought it was no big deal for people to gain weight with aging, assuring him that it was a natural part of the process. Banting refused to accept that, though, which makes sense given the increasing pressure he must have felt: his size was suddenly putting him at odds with the classist, racist, and sexist ideas circulating in Western culture about how a well-to-do white man "should" look. Eventually he found a doctor who agreed to put him on an austere, experimental diet.

In 1864 Banting published a pamphlet titled *Letter on Corpulence: Addressed to the Public*, outlining the diet his doctor had prescribed and explaining how he'd apparently overcome his own weight struggles, including detailed logs of changes in his weight over time. The pamphlet was so popular that it sold out and had to be reprinted multiple times, and eventually it was published as a book of the same name—the first modern diet book, a trailblazer in terms of taking diets out of the realm of medical therapy and into the domain of self-help.[26] The book was a sensation in Europe and the U.S., and it was covered widely in the press.

Banting's introduction reads a lot like many of today's diet books, old-timey language aside: "Of all the parasites that affect humanity I do not know of, nor can I imagine, any more distressing than that of Obesity, and, having just emerged from a very long probation in this affliction, I am desirous of circulating my humble knowledge and experience for the benefit of my fellow man, with an earnest hope it may lead to the same comfort and happiness I now feel under the extraordinary change."[27] In other words, "I got thin and it changed my life! Here's how you can do it, too."

He also discussed the weight-related stigma he'd experienced in adulthood: "I am confident no man laboring under obesity can be quite insensible to the sneers and remarks of the cruel and injudicious in public assemblies, public vehicles, or the ordinary street traffic; nor to the annoyance of finding no adequate space in a public assembly if he should seek amusement or need refreshment, and therefore he naturally keeps away as much as possible from places where he is likely to be made the object of taunts and remarks of others." Just as it is today, fatness was increasingly demonized in Banting's time, and larger-bodied people were the targets of exclusion and derision. It's no wonder he wanted to escape that fate. The diet he outlined in the pamphlet—which came to be known as the Banting diet—was low in carbs and high in meat and fat, sort of like a proto-Atkins diet (but with a lot more alcohol, on the order of six glasses a day, apparently to help counteract the constipating effects of eating almost nothing but meat).

Banting's book, with its obsessive logging of body weights, helped ignite a cultural obsession with the scale. When the book was first published, scales were a novelty item in the U.S. People would weigh themselves at regional fairs and exhibitions, where manufacturers encouraged attendees to step on giant platform scales designed for agricultural and industrial uses—a publicity stunt meant to show just how accurate these scales were. They weren't really made for weighing people, and that was the fun of it. Banting's attention to weight helped change all that, creating a demand for scales that were more widely available and more finely calibrated for the human body.

The first human scales were sold to health-care facilities and were too cumbersome and expensive for use by most people. Then a technological innovation appeared that suddenly allowed people to start weighing themselves regularly: the "penny scale," a coin-operated platform-style scale that was introduced in the U.S. in 1885 and quickly spread throughout the country.[28] Soon there were penny scales everywhere—in drugstores, train stations, grocery stores, and eventually even banks, movie theaters, and office buildings. The scales spread in part because they were so profitable for their manufacturers and owner-operators, bringing in hundreds of thousands of dollars of revenue over the years. The proliferation of penny scales also fanned the flames of people's emerging, painful self-consciousness about weight—although interestingly, at first the chief concern among women was being too thin, not too fat.

Despite the emerging cultural view of fatness as a mark of "uncivilized" status, for most of the Victorian era (1837–1901) it had been considered the height of beauty and refinement for women to be plump, pale, hourglass-shaped (with the help of corsets), and swathed in layers of poufed fabric—signs that their husbands could afford to feed them well and keep them away from manual labor.[29] The Victorian preference for larger bodies clearly had nothing to do with feminism, and these beauty standards were also bound up with classism and racism, where looking beautiful meant looking rich and white. Women were still being oppressed, but not yet by an impossibly thin beauty ideal. Instead, doctors encouraged people to *gain* weight, and photographers considered hollow cheekbones and prominent collarbones to be defects. Actress Lillian Russell, the great beauty of the era whose voluptuous shape was widely admired, would fall in the "obese" category on today's body mass index chart, whereas thinner actresses were publicly mocked. The Victorian beauty standard was about taking up *more* space, not less.

The vogue for larger bodies among women would soon change, though. Print media was on the rise, reaching more and more people, and it became the perfect vehicle for disseminating a new image of what women "should" look like in this increasingly anti-fat culture: the Gibson Girl. Created by artist Charles Dana Gibson in 1890 for *Life* magazine, the Gibson Girl was a pen-and-ink drawing of a young, white, well-to-do woman who bucked some Victorian trends in a way that felt fresh and exciting at the time.[30] Like the Victorian ideal, the Gibson Girl was still hourglass-shaped and narrow-waisted—impossibly so, since she was a *drawing* and didn't have the pesky human constraint of internal organs—but with a more athletic body type that matched her novel hobbies: tennis, croquet, bicycling, and other high-society sports.[31] Instead of being wrapped up in layers of voluminous fabric, she wore less-fussy clothes more suitable for movement. Gibson created numerous versions of the character for *Life*, and they soon became a sensation. Other magazines clamored for his illustrations, and Gibson Girls started to be used in advertisements to sell everything from soap to vacation getaways.

The Gibson Girl was hailed as a welcome departure from the confines of Victorian womanhood. She was the New Woman! writers declared. She showed that women could actually do stuff! But her look was a pure fabrication—basically the nineteenth-century version of a Barbie doll, or the Photoshopped lady-bots we see in magazines today. And just like those modern-day images, the Gibson Girl made women want to do and buy whatever it took to get that look. As Laura Fraser wrote in her 1997 book *Losing It: False Hopes and Fat Profits in the Diet Industry,* "Women would buy products advertised by a Gibson Girl in the hope that some of her beauty, social position, and vitality would rub off on them." The practice of using aspirational images of thin white ladies in advertising was born, ushering in generations of women who felt inadequate by comparison.

Women and the Thin Ideal

From the Gibson Girl onward, advertising and fashion continued to put the squeeze on middle-class women with an increasingly thin beauty ideal. By the early 1900s, magazines such as *Life* and daily newspapers across the country overflowed with advertisements for weight-loss products, including compression garments that supposedly reduced fat through pressure (emphasis on *supposedly*) and diet pills that contained arsenic, industrial toxins, thyroid extract, and even tapeworms.[32] In 1908 a high-end French designer created a revolutionary sheath dress that became fashionable among society ladies, and that style started to trickle down to the masses in the 1910s.[33] Then a daring young designer named Coco Chanel refined the dress silhouette by dropping its waistline and raising its hemline, and the flapper dress was born. It went along with a whole flapper culture,

epitomized by late-night jazz shows, cigarettes, sexual liberation, and above all youth.

The whole thing was a flagrant rebellion against Victorian
values—and that included a repudiation of Victorian beauty
ideals, going much further than the Gibson Girl had gone. But
in many ways the new flapper aesthetic was even more constricting. Whereas Victorian women dressed to create an hourglass
shape, flappers' clothes were all straight, slim lines, and women
had to bind their breasts and restrict their food intake to fit into
them without any curves peeking out. In an era that increasingly worshipped youthfulness, having the body of a grown (cisgender) woman was profoundly uncool. (It's worth noting here
that although the flapper beauty ideal was significantly thinner
than any American ideal that had come before, by today's standards flappers would still be considered "refreshingly real."
That's a testament to how beauty standards have continued to
narrow over the years since diet culture was born.) By the 1920s,
women had traded in the literal corsets of the Victorian era for
what Fraser calls the "inner corset" of self-imposed starvation.

Women did legitimately gain tremendous freedom and
political power in this era, particularly in 1920 with the adop-
tion of the Nineteenth Amendment, which gave women the
right to vote. But the diet industry also took things to the next
level that decade, bringing a glut of new products to the market.
Advertisers ingeniously paired images of slim flappers with
pitches for products such as scales, laxatives, and "reducing
soaps" that claimed to wash away fat. And, of course, restrictive
diets became another product in the mix. Companies were
scrambling to sell supposed solutions to the problem of being
"overweight"—a word that had not been used to describe people until 1899.[34] Though flappers were genuinely more at liberty
to come and go and be in the world than their Victorian mothers, this younger generation was in many ways far more restricted
by unrealistic beauty standards.

That's probably no coincidence. As feminist writer Naomi Wolf argues, the times in history when women have made the greatest political gains—getting the vote, gaining reproductive freedom, securing the right to work outside the home—have also been moments when standards for "ideal" beauty became significantly thinner and the pressure on women to adhere to those standards increased. Wolf explains that this serves both to distract women from their growing political power and to assuage the fears of people who don't want the old patriarchal system to change—because if women are busy trying to shrink themselves, they won't have the time or energy to shake things up. It's hard to smash the patriarchy on an empty stomach, or with a head full of food and body concerns, and that's exactly the point of diet culture. Or as Wolf famously put it: "Dieting is the most potent political sedative in women's history; a quietly mad population is a tractable one."[35] Today, dieting—which includes participating in "plans," "protocols," "lifestyle changes," "resets," and other diets that claim not to be diets, as we'll discuss in Chapter 2—continues to have this sedative function for women, but also increasingly for people of all genders. It keeps us too hungry, too fixated on our bodies, and too caught up in the minutiae of our eating regimens to focus our energies on changing the world.

The propaganda used in opposing women's suffrage is a perfect example of how beauty and body-size standards get harnessed in efforts to undercut women's power. In the early twentieth century, being fat was seen as a sign of lower evolutionary status, as was failing or refusing to adhere to binary gender roles and beauty standards. The anti-suffrage movement exploited these beliefs in posters, ads, and political cartoons that portrayed suffragists as fat, masculine, and angry, with the aim of dissuading women from joining the movement.[36] On a 1910 cover of the humor magazine *Judge*, for example, a large-bodied, masculine-looking woman stands in a kitchen, surrounded by pots and pans, staring menacingly at the viewer with angry, wild eyes. She holds a gigantic rolling pin in one muscular hand and a huge spoon in the other—the implication being that she's going to clock you if she doesn't get her way. The caption reads "Speaker of the House," lampooning the woman's effort to participate in public life when clearly her proper place is in the kitchen. Her looks imply that the desire for power and rights has turned her into an "uncivilized" creature, a monster. The message of the cartoon was clear: Suffragists are terrifying; don't be one of them. (That line of rhetoric has continued to this day, in the stereotype of feminists as angry, "man-hating" killjoys.)

Meanwhile, first-wave feminists themselves played a role in the demonization of fatness. Women's-rights activists in the early 1900s fought back against the anti-suffrage propaganda by issuing their own messaging that portrayed suffragists as thin, white, and beautiful—and their opponents as fat, "uncivilized," and ugly.[37] These early feminists aimed to bolster their case that women were sufficiently "evolved" to deserve the right to vote, rather than questioning the premise that people in certain kinds of bodies deserved rights and others didn't. Though of course it's great that women eventually won the right to vote, these early suffragists' tactics also helped entrench other forms of oppression, including the racist and sizeist beauty ideal.

Science and Medicine Jump on the Diet-Culture Train

The last major piece in the root system of diet culture is the emergence of health rationales for weight stigma. Whereas doctors in the early to mid-1800s had generally seen weight gain and fatness as a natural part of the aging process, by the early 1900s physicians were starting to get on board with the idea that weight loss was the way to go. That wasn't because of scientific evidence in favor of weight loss—there really wasn't any to speak of at the time—but rather because of the already strong cultural bias against fatness. The fad for thinness influenced doctors' thinking, which in turn affected the advice they gave their patients and any scientific articles they published.[38] Contrary to what modern-day diet culture would have you believe, cultural fatphobia pre-dated any health arguments about body size. It's no surprise that physicians got caught up in this anti-fat trend, because doctors are people, too—subject to the whims of fashion and culture just like the rest of us. (That's equally true today, by the way; doctors are just as much citizens of twenty-first-century diet culture as we all are.)

Turn-of-the-century physicians were also subject to pressure from their patients, who from the early 1900s often came in asking for weight-loss advice. Some doctors were annoyed by this behavior—seeing it as mere vanity that took them away from addressing more serious health issues—but eventually most physicians did what any business owner does in the face of overwhelming demand: give the people what they want. By the 1920s, almost every medical office had a scale.[39]

Doctors were also influenced by the burgeoning life- and health-insurance industries. Around the turn of the twentieth century, insurance companies started using height-weight tables inspired by the work of a Belgian astronomer and statistician named Adolphe Quetelet—whose Quetelet index is now known as the body mass index, or BMI—to categorize people as "normal weight," "overweight," and "underweight," with "normal" being considered ideal. There were (and still are) many problems with that equation: for one, Quetelet developed it in the 1830s as a way to test whether the laws of probability could be applied to human beings at the population level. It was created as a statistical exercise, not a medical instrument, and was never intended for clinical use. Quetelet also developed his equation using an exclusively white, European population—the people in his environment—which means that it doesn't account for differences in average body size in other ethnic groups.[40]

None of these flaws stopped the insurance companies from using variations on the Quetelet index, though. In 1899 the president of the Association of Life Insurance Medical Directors of America presented some preliminary data from several insurance companies, stating that "from our mortality records the overweights are clearly less desirable than either the normal or the underweights."[41] These records were based almost exclusively on wealthy white men, but modern-day data from much larger, more representative samples shows that "the overweights" actually have the *lowest* mortality risk of any group on the BMI chart.[42] The BMI is also notoriously imprecise; it can't tell you anything about a person's body composition, nor can it accurately predict their health outcomes. Indeed, many researchers over the years have recommended that BMI be discarded as an outdated and ineffective tool for measuring health.[43]

Drawing on those dubious data from their insurance pools, insurers began bombarding doctors with literature on the supposed risks of higher weights.[44] Insurance companies didn't know why people in larger bodies seemed to have a higher mortality risk, or what the cause-and-effect relationship was, if any, between weight and health. But obviously money was at stake, and the culture had already been shifting in an anti-fat direction, so it was fairly easy for the theory that higher weights caused worse health to take root in the medical community.

That fatphobia was further entrenched in the 1910s, when World War I caused international food shortages that radically altered Americans' relationship with food.[45] The government created an agency called the Food Administration and charged it with heading up voluntary food-conservation efforts as well as "rationalizing" national eating habits—creating rules and order in a domain where emotion, tradition, and pleasure had long reigned supreme. The stakes were high, given the very real food crisis going on in Europe at the time, and so this American food-reform movement became something of a moral crusade. The Food Administration's slogan, "Victory over Ourselves," was meant as a reminder that self-discipline with food was a moral imperative that would ensure the survival of the republic. In this context where moralized rhetoric about food reached (or even surpassed) Ancient Greek levels, people began to see fatness as evidence of moral failure, an outward sign that a person supposedly couldn't control their inner appetites.

The emerging field of nutrition science quickly became entangled in this fatphobic, moralistic food-reform movement, as food administrators used advances in the nutrition field to claim the authority to tell people what to eat. As historian Helen Zoe Veit writes, "The wartime food conservation campaign helped popularize nutrition science, and its popularity was speeded, not slowed, by the moralism embedded in it." In other words, the fact that nutrition science was tied up with ideas about morality was a feature, not a bug. And that would help shape the field for decades to come (spoiler alert: including today).

Diet Culture in Full Force

With all those roots firmly in place, diet culture took hold with shocking force in the American mainstream in the 1920s and '30s, across racial and socioeconomic lines.[46] In these early days, diets were all remarkably similar in their reliance on the concept of "willpower"—another term that had entered the American lexicon in the late nineteenth century. Fatness was now widely considered a failure of the will, and blatantly bigoted anti-fat sentiments became commonplace in diet books, popular culture, and the medical community. In the 1920s people took up self-harming methods such as smoking cigarettes and fasting to try to lose weight, sometimes urged on by doctors. In

the 1930s physicians recommended diets that had people subsisting on little more than fruit and milk, and gyms sprang up
with those weird vibrating belts that supposedly "loosened" fat
so it could melt away. (Nope—not effective.) Interestingly, the
Depression didn't put an end to the vogue for dieting; people
remained obsessed with getting thin, but now they were doing it
on a budget.[47]

Diet pills were also all the rage, starting in the 1930s with
Benzedrine, then progressing in the 1940s to amphetamines
(aka speed), which were given freely to World War II soldiers to
help them stay awake in combat and became popular as weight-
loss aids thereafter. Gyms and fitness became more popular
over the ensuing decades, and the 1950s saw the rise of televised
"calisthenics" classes designed to help people shrink their bodies. Despite the public's apparent interest in health, the market
for diet pills was still booming: by 1970, 8 percent of all prescriptions written in the U.S. were for amphetamines, and at least a
fifth of those prescriptions were explicitly for weight loss, even
though the American Medical Association (AMA) had issued a
public warning against using these drugs for dieting as early as
1943.

Meanwhile, in the 1950s the market for bariatric surgery was
born. The first such surgery was performed in 1953 at the University of Minnesota.[48] At that time physicians generally saw bariatric surgery as an elective treatment, to be used only in rare
cases—because, you know, amputating a healthy stomach is not
exactly a normal thing to do.[49] Doctors didn't think of the surgery
as a "medically necessary" intervention with a potential market
of millions of people, the way they do today. But one physician—
a bariatric surgeon named Howard Payne—saw things differently. In an effort to expand his practice, Payne coined the term
morbid obesity. It was an ingenious way to frame bariatric surgery
as a necessary and even lifesaving intervention, because labeling
people's body size as *morbid* makes it sound like they're about to

drop dead. By creating a new class of larger bodies that were supposedly near death because of their size, Payne made the strictures of diet culture a little more oppressive.

Most people still weren't opting for surgery, though; instead, they turned in increasing numbers to group dieting programs. Take Off Pounds Sensibly (TOPS) was founded in 1948, Overeaters Anonymous in 1960, and Weight Watchers in 1961, the latter when housewife Jean Nidetch began hosting informal meetings with her dieting friends in her living room.[50] Nidetch's experience with yo-yo dieting over the years had led her to believe she couldn't stick to any diet because of "emotional overeating," and she thought the solution was likewise emotional: support groups, motivational speeches, and even weight-loss camps designed to increase people's likelihood of staying on the diet (which at the time was a very '60s regime that demonized dietary fat). The concept of emotional overeating was very of-the-moment, too: it originated with psychiatrist Hilde Bruch, a researcher who studied larger-bodied children and believed that "childhood obesity" was caused by mothers who overfed their kids, substituting food for affection.

Bruch's arguments about the origins of children's body size were later debunked, but at the time her ideas were hot. They became part of the popular consciousness in the '60s as they were disseminated by other researchers, the media, and the diet and food industries—which, of course, had a vested interest in framing diet failure as an emotional issue, rather than a defect in the diets themselves. (To this day, that framing often keeps people stuck in the futile cycle of yo-yo dieting, as we'll discuss in Chapter 6.)

Nidetch's portrayal of diet failure as an emotional issue struck a cultural chord, helping propel Weight Watchers to quick success: she incorporated the business in 1963 and by 1968 five million people had enrolled, with hundreds of franchise locations around the world. Dozens of other group-dieting programs that emphasized emotions came on the scene in the '60s, including many that riffed on the "Anonymous" name, among them Eaters Anonymous, Gluttons Anonymous, and Fatties Anonymous.[51]

Counterculture and Contradictions

The same year that Weight Watchers was incorporated, Betty Friedan's seminal book *The Feminine Mystique* was published—a searing critique of the cultural norms that kept too many women unhappily stuck in the role of the '50s suburban housewife. The book deeply resonated with millions of people and is widely credited with launching second-wave feminism in the United States. Yet as with women's suffrage in 1920, this new wave of feminism was quickly followed by the emergence of a thinner-than-ever beauty standard. In 1966 a waiflike, sixteen-year-old British model nicknamed Twiggy ushered in the thinnest beauty ideal to date. She became both the world's first supermodel and a symbol of a newly unattainable standard for most grown women.

Meanwhile, food and the body were becoming battlegrounds in new social movements. The 1960s and '70s saw the rise of civil rights, gay liberation, feminism, the environmental movement, antiwar protests, and other forms of countercultural rebellion against the status quo. People were recognizing that "the personal is political"—that is, that making conscious choices in their own lives could help change the system. They started to see food as a way to take a political stand for social and environmental justice and against the interests of big business, capitalism, white supremacy, and the patriarchy. These countercultural ideas about food were intended to oppose many of the same oppressive forces that create pressure on people to meet impossible standards of beauty. But as we'll see shortly, diet culture eventually twisted the ideals of the '60s and '70s food movement to its own ends.

Around the same time that other important social-justice movements were gaining ground, the fat-liberation movement was born. Just as these other movements advocated for rights and recognition for various marginalized groups—women, people of color, gay people, people with disabilities—fat-liberation activists fought for the rights of people whom society deemed "overweight" or "obese," seeking to reclaim even the word *fat* from a society intent on pathologizing it. Fat-liberation groups including, most notably, the Fat Underground worked to raise awareness about the scientific evidence against dieting and intentional weight loss, which eventually caught the attention of some mainstream health professionals and academics.

Still, mainstream diet culture from the 1970s through the 1990s reached a fever pitch, with wildly contradictory claims about nutrition contributing to an ever-more-chaotic national relationship with food. The market for dieting grew rapidly during this period because more people from more diverse backgrounds— including men, people of color, and the elderly—were trying to control their weight and believed they were "overweight" (even if the BMI chart said otherwise).[52] The result was a proliferation of new nutrition trends and fad diets—almost too many to mention, but here are some of the highlights:

In 1972 cardiologist Robert Atkins published his bestselling book *Dr. Atkins' Diet Revolution,* arguing that the best diet was high in fat and protein and extremely low in carbohydrates; the prevailing scientific wisdom at the time vilified dietary fat, however, and in 1977 the federal government officially endorsed a low-fat diet in its Dietary Goals for the United States.[53] (Cue explosion in the market for low-fat diet foods.) In 1983 the weight-loss clinic Jenny Craig opened its doors—the same year that singer Karen Carpenter died of anorexia. In 1988 Oprah Winfrey famously dragged a wagon full of fat across the stage of her TV studio, saying it was the amount of weight she'd lost on a commercial diet that billed itself as a "medically supervised" alternative to typical diets. In 1992 a National Institutes of Health panel of weight-science experts concluded that diets don't work, and that the vast majority of people who've intentionally lost weight regain most or all of it within five years.[54] Oprah was already among that majority by then; she says that in 1992 she was the heaviest she's ever been,[55] a highly visible example of how fleeting weight loss really is for most people. Yet the same year, Atkins reissued his low-carb manifesto as *Dr. Atkins' New Diet Revolution,* and the deadly weight-loss drug fen-phen hit the market (only to be banned five years later because it was found to cause heart-valve defects). And in 1994 the Guide to Nutrition Labeling and Education Act took effect in the U.S., requiring manufacturers to post nutrition information on nearly all food packaging—which meant that now people could check the amount of calories, carbs, or fat in food for themselves, becoming even more obsessive in their dieting.

The *Washington Post* reported in 1995 that Americans were "fatter than ever before," and that one of the leading theories why was because "a decade of dieting mania has actually made people fatter."[56] The article didn't explain exactly how diets can lead to weight gain, but it did point out that most diets don't produce weight loss that lasts more than two or three years, and that dieting often causes people to become obsessed with food. A doctor from Baylor College of Medicine in Houston was quoted as saying, "The more you diet, the worse it gets" and "To hell with the weight. The scale is to the dieter what the roulette wheel is to a chronic gambler. Get away from that mentality. Get away from the obsession with body image." Was this the beginning of the end for the diet industry? Were the medical field and the general public finally starting to wake up and realize that dieting was a colossal waste of time that failed to deliver on the results it promised?

Not so much. By the mid-1990s, 44 percent of women and 29 percent of men reported that they were trying to lose weight, up from roughly 14 percent of women and 7 percent of men between 1950 and 1966.[57] It wasn't just people in larger bodies trying to lose weight, either; 37 percent of the women and 11 percent of the men trying to lose weight in the mid-'90s were in the "normal" BMI category. Since the 1960s, every decade has had its whistle-blowers calling out the problematic nature of dieting and the thin ideal, yet diet culture is still going strong today—a testament to its ability to constantly reinvent itself by morphing into increasingly subtle, sneaky forms that elude detection and allow the Life Thief to maintain its hold on us.

In 1999 Atkins reissued his book a third time. Again it became a bestseller, followed by numerous other low-carb diet books such as *The Zone* and *The South Beach Diet.* They were nothing new—this style of diet went back to the days of William Banting, remember—but at this particular moment in history they caused a revolution in the public's relationship with carbohydrates. Low-carb products began crowding out fat-free foods on the shelves, and a new widespread panic about carbs upended decades of low-fat domination.

The Making of the "Obesity Epidemic"

In 1998 millions of Americans became "overweight" and "obese" *literally* overnight. It wasn't because they had epically binged before going to bed—contrary to what diet culture would have you believe, a binge won't make you suddenly larger. It was something much more bureaucratic: The National Institutes of Health (NIH), the U.S. federal agency in charge of setting the official BMI categories for American guidelines, released a report changing its thresholds for what it considered "overweight" and "obese." People suddenly moved into new, higher BMI categories without having gained any weight whatsoever, simply because the cutoffs had changed.

The NIH is ostensibly an unbiased organization devoted to public health, yet the reality of how these cutoffs were established is quite political, as we can see by tracing their origins. The NIH based them on a report that the World Health Organization (WHO) had put out two years before—which, in turn, was primarily written by another organization called the International Obesity Task Force (IOTF). And the IOTF was funded largely by two pharmaceutical companies that make weight-loss drugs: Hoffmann–La Roche and Abbott Laboratories.[58] The IOTF's purpose was to lobby for and create science that supports the interests of the pharmaceutical industry—and, of course, lowering BMI cutoffs so that millions more Americans think they have a "weight problem" is definitely in the interest of pharmaceutical companies selling weight-loss drugs.

Individual "obesity experts" involved in changing these cutoffs also had deep ties to the diet industry. For example, the chair of the NIH panel on "obesity" was a doctor and researcher named Xavier Pi-Sunyer, who has served on the advisory board or as a paid consultant for drug and weight-loss companies including Wyeth-Ayerst Laboratories (makers of lethal fen-phen), Eli Lilly Pharmaceuticals, Genentech, and Weight Watchers International.[59] Pi-Sunyer was also a member of the WHO panel that lowered the BMI cutoffs in 1995, as well as a member of the IOTF. As political scientist J. Eric Oliver wrote of these cozy relationships in his 2005 book, *Fat Politics,* "It is difficult to find any major figure in the field of obesity research…who does not have some type of financial tie to a pharmaceutical or weight-loss company."

Why does it matter if researchers have these financial ties, you might ask. It matters because industry funding has been shown to significantly and substantially affect the outcomes of research. A 2016 review of research on artificial sweeteners, for example, found that studies financed by food-industry sources were seventeen times more likely to have favorable results than those funded by non-industry sources.[60] When you're being paid by a company to research its product, you're probably going to want to produce results that keep the bosses happy.

Aside from the incentives they were getting from the diet industry, "obesity" researchers had their own stake in lowering the BMI thresholds: it increased the perceived importance of their work, giving them more opportunities to get funding as well as increased power and prestige.[61] Sure enough, soon after the 1998 NIH report was released, the budgets for "obesity" programs at the NIH and the Centers for Disease Control (CDC) increased substantially. At the NIH alone, funding for "obesity" research jumped from about $50 million in 1993 to more than $400 million by 2004 (or more than $308 million in 1993 dollars).[62] By adding nearly forty million people to the numbers supposedly at risk because of their weight, the NIH elevated "obesity" to a level of public-health importance it had never had before.

That laid the groundwork for the concept of an "obesity epidemic," but it wasn't enough on its own to make the idea spread in the viral way that it ultimately did. What really brought the notion to its tipping point was a small but mighty vector: a Power-Point presentation. It was based on the work of a researcher named William Dietz (like *diets* with a *z*—you can't make this stuff up), who was then a director of the CDC's Division for Nutrition and Physical Activity.[63] Dietz was heavily invested in promulgating the belief that "obesity," beyond being associated with undesirable health outcomes, was a disease unto itself—and one that was spreading. People, in his view, were getting unhealthier because they were getting fatter, and the public-health community needed to do something about it.

This was a controversial point of view in the late 1990s. It had started to gain traction in certain corners of the medical field in the 1960s and '70s, when "obesity" began to be medical-ized.[64] But Dietz's opinion wasn't yet widespread, and many of his fellow researchers at the CDC didn't see "obesity" as a real problem.[65] The data tracking the BMIs of Americans over the years just didn't seem all that remarkable to Dietz's colleagues, even though there was a slight upward trend in weights over time. But then Dietz and another CDC scientist named Ali Mok-dad came up with a novel idea: instead of presenting the data in boring tables, the way most statistical data is shown, they would create a series of maps showing the percentage of people in each state who fell into the "obese" BMI category, and arrange them as a slideshow. The maps were color-coded so that the states with the lowest rates of "obesity" (below 10 percent) appeared in light blue; those with higher rates appeared in darker blues; and those with rates above 20 percent appeared in red.[66] The first "obesity" map, showing rates in 1985, is largely white—indicating that there was no data for many states—but the states that do have data are all light or medium blue, with no red in sight. As you flip through the slides, year by year, the col-ors on the map start to fill in, and the blues start to darken. The map for 1994 is a mix of medium and dark blues, with the darker hues concentrated in the South and much of the Midwest. By 1998 it's mostly dark blue, with seven states in red. The effect is striking.

The maps created a powerful sense of an epidemic spread-ing across the country, and they convinced anyone who saw them that Americans' increasing body size wasn't a neutral fact (like the increase in average height that happened during that same period) but a genuine epidemic. As Dietz explained to *Fat Politics* author Oliver, "After people have seen the maps, we no longer have to discuss whether a problem with obesity exists. These maps have shifted the discussion from whether a problem exists to what we should do about the epidemic."[67]

The real problem is that these maps are incredibly misleading. For one thing, a weight gain of only a few pounds can tip someone from the "overweight" category into the "obese" category. So it wasn't that Americans were gaining huge amounts of weight and ending up "obese"; it was that people already in larger bodies gained, on average, a small amount of weight (we're talking a single-digit number of pounds here) and crossed into the maligned "obese" category. The maps are also based on the *percentage* of people in each state who fall into the "obese" category, rather than on the overall number in each state — and as is painfully clear in every U.S. presidential election, states with comparatively tiny populations can have a major effect on the color of the map. While it might seem like entire swaths of the country are becoming "obese," it's really just that large, rural states are making it look that way. Moreover, poverty is associated with larger body size; as Oliver points out, "The reason the first 'outbreaks' of obesity were in Mississippi, Alabama, and West Virginia was not because they were near some viral source but because these states are largely rural and poor." It was wrong to categorize larger body size as an "epidemic" for many reasons (including the fact that it increases weight stigma—which, as we'll discuss in Chapter 5, is dangerous for your health), but the biggest reason is that it simply wasn't true. The average weight in the U.S. may have crept up a little from 1985 to 1998, but that was hardly a mass outbreak of disease. Instead, the "obesity epidemic" is really a moral panic that has a lot more to do with diet culture's skewed beliefs about weight than with any actual threat to public health.[68]

Another extremely important factor that never gets discussed in relation to the "obesity epidemic" is dieting; as we'll discuss in Chapter 3, intentional weight-loss efforts have been shown to cause long-term weight *gain* for up to two-thirds of the people who embark on them. So if the national average weight was creeping up over the years, it's a good bet that dieting was at least partly responsible for the increase. Indeed, as we discussed, the 1970s through 1990s were particularly intense decades for diet culture, with widespread concern and confusion about the healthiest way to eat and an exponential rise in the number of people trying to lose weight. Given this increasing national panic about body size, it's really no wonder people were getting heavier. (I'm by no means painting this weight gain as a bad thing, by the way—weight is a morally neutral trait, and there's nothing wrong with you if you gain weight or live in a larger body.) Yet rather than acknowledging that dieting leads to weight gain over the long term, diet culture loves to point the finger at other factors—the latest one being processed food and the food industry. As we'll discuss in Chapter 9, no good scientific evidence exists that eating so-called "processed" (or "highly palatable") food causes significant weight gain or poor health outcomes. But as you'll see in Chapter 3, there *is* strong evidence that intentional weight-loss efforts result in long-term weight gain for a large percentage of people.

The dubiousness of the maps' claims didn't stop the idea of an "obesity epidemic" from spreading. In 1998 Dietz posted the slides on the CDC website, where anyone could download them. Other government officials soon picked them up; researchers and academics wrote about them in scientific publications. As Oliver says of himself and other researchers who drew attention to the maps, "We were, in effect, carriers of the disease model, transmitting it across a much larger population."[69] Soon health reporters at major news outlets, who tend to closely follow what's being reported in scientific journals, started to parrot the phrase *obesity epidemic,* which led to an explosion in news coverage using that language. By 1999 some 50 articles referred to this supposed epidemic; by 2000 the number had more than doubled, to 107; and by 2004 there were nearly 700, an exponential growth. Thus the *idea* of an "obesity epidemic" spread like an epidemic itself. One could argue that this was just a matter of aesthetics—a linguistic trend similar to every scandal being dubbed "X-gate" after Watergate—but in fact the choice to frame body size as an epidemic had a very real, very harmful impact on people's lives, as we'll discuss in the next chapter.

Today the prevailing view is that "obesity" is one of the biggest, baddest killers around, and that the problem with fatness is not about looks but about health. By 2013 the AMA had classified "obesity" as a disease, ignoring the recommendations of its own committee devoted to studying the issue.[70] That committee had ruled that "obesity" should *not* be considered a disease, primarily because of the difficulty in defining it and especially given that BMI—the measure usually used to assess "obesity"—is deeply flawed. That argument apparently didn't hold water with higher-ups at the association, perhaps because drug companies and surgeons stood to gain so much financially from the "disease" label, which would increase insurance reimbursements for treatment. Ironically, one reason the AMA cited in favor of applying the "disease" label is that it would reduce the stigma of "obesity." But as we'll discuss in the next chapter, that framing only exacerbates weight stigma.

As you can see from this quick trip through the history of diet culture, it's very much a system of oppression, with its roots in racist, sexist beliefs about food and bodies. Over time, those roots have become increasingly obscured by the ever-changing, ever-subtler, and seemingly benign ways that diet culture shows up in the world. Although some of that obscuring occurs simply because diet culture has become the default point of view in Western society—the water we've all been swimming in since birth, without realizing it—there are other, more nefarious reasons why it can be hard to recognize diet culture for the Life Thief it really is. In fact concealing diet culture's true roots is a deliberate move that the diet industry uses to keep itself afloat, as you're about to see.

CHAPTER 2

A Diet by Another Name

In 2008 sociologist Abigail Saguy enlisted a promising undergraduate student to help research her book *What's Wrong with Fat?*[1] The student—Saguy calls her Liz, a pseudonym—was tasked with helping Saguy collect and catalogue news reports about two conflicting scientific studies: one from 2004 that found being in the "overweight" and "obese" BMI categories was associated with hundreds of thousands of excess deaths, and a second from 2005 showing that being in the "overweight" category is associated with *fewer* deaths than being in the "normal-weight" category.

Liz started by collecting reports about the 2004 study. As she made her way through article after article painting fatness as a public-health crisis of the highest order, Liz started to feel worse and worse about her own body. She had managed to make it to college without ever having gone on a diet—a rarity for any woman living in diet culture, and likely due to the privilege of having a BMI in the "normal" range. But after cataloguing all those fearmongering news reports about the "obesity epidemic," Liz started worrying that her weight was too high and went on her first diet.

When she told Saguy what had happened, "I was pretty disturbed," Saguy says. She promptly told Liz about the findings of the 2005 study (Liz hadn't started that phase of the research yet), which showed that "obesity" is actually associated with a lower mortality risk than "underweight" and roughly equal to that of "normal weight." Saguy had Liz start collecting news reports about the second study instead. Once she'd finished that research, Liz returned to Saguy's office visibly more relaxed. She said she'd stopped her diet and was feeling better about her body. Saguy had initially been looking into how media reports framed each of these studies, but Liz's experience made her curious: How many other people have reactions like this when reading news reports about the "obesity epidemic"? And in general, how does framing fatness as a public-health issue affect our perceptions of people in larger bodies?

Saguy and a team of researchers designed a series of tests to find out. The results were striking: across multiple experiments with thousands of participants, reports framing "obesity" as a public-health crisis and a matter of personal responsibility led to greater anti-fat prejudice in general, and to a willingness to discriminate against people with "obese" BMIs in the workplace, as well as more support for charging these people higher rates for health insurance.[2] "The finding that even just reading an article about the 'obesity epidemic' increases expressed stigma is very robust," Saguy says. She explains that these results are consistent with other research showing that people are more likely to express discriminatory views about fatness when they believe that body size is a matter of willpower, because when the argument is framed in that way, people feel more justified in expressing their anti-fat prejudices and less need to suppress them.[3]

Although the "fat is unhealthy" articles in Saguy's experiment didn't seem to affect readers' personal body image in the way she had anticipated based on Liz's experience,* the "public-health

---

* Saguy says this might be because people in the experiment weren't asked to wade through dozens and dozens of these articles, as Liz was. Or it might be because Liz had been "unusually sheltered" from these kinds of articles before starting the project, given that she was in the "normal" BMI category and had never dieted before.

crisis" framing has an even greater social impact: It increases the expression of discrimination against an already marginalized group of people. It creates social injustice and causes harm on a collective level.

What if reports framing "obesity" as a health risk also included the message that it's unacceptable to discriminate against people based on their body size—would that change the outcome? No dice. When Saguy and her colleagues showed study participants articles that included anti-stigma messaging along with information on the supposed health risks of "obesity," the participants' anti-fat attitudes held steady.[4] Saguy explains that this is likely because people are so inundated with "obesity epidemic" rhetoric and other fatphobic ideas in our culture that tacking anti-discrimination messages onto the usual health arguments isn't enough to change their minds. Arguing that "obesity" is bad for people's health still reinforces weight stigma, even if you try to make those arguments in a kinder, gentler way. Instead, we shouldn't be framing "obesity" as a cause of poor health outcomes at all—both because the idea of an "obesity epidemic" was largely fabricated by people with a vested interest in the weight-loss industry and because weight *stigma* and the pressure to diet may explain any correlations we see between larger body size and poor health outcomes.

A 2018 study by another researcher extended Saguy's findings, showing that moralized arguments about health in general—including "obesity epidemic" rhetoric and value judgments about "healthy lifestyles"—are associated with greater stigmatization of people who deviate from the supposed picture of health, greater exclusion of these people from society, and lower levels of social cohesion.[5] "Governments' good intentions in persuading entire populations to live more healthily might come at a substantial cost, especially when the discourse highlights morality," the study concludes. Thus, framing "obesity" and "healthy lifestyles" as matters of public-health importance, personal responsibility, and morality has the unintended consequence of creating and exacerbating stigma against people in larger bodies. And as we'll discuss in later chapters, that stigma *in and of itself* is harmful to people's health.

It's not just newspaper articles and public-health officials that contribute to the stigmatizing of larger bodies, though. In the twenty-first century, that stigma shows up in all sorts of unexpected places, often cloaked as concern for health and well-being. The current cultural obsession with "wellness" presents itself as an alternative to diet culture, but really it's just the Life Thief's latest iteration—a diet by another name. People generally think they're doing the right thing by educating themselves on habits to promote health, and that isn't the issue per se. Hell, I'm a health professional—I value health and well-being, too, for my clients as well as for my loved ones and myself. The problem is that diet culture has framed *its* version of health and wellness as both a moral obligation and the be-all and end-all of life, and millions of us have bought into that belief—to the point where it's doing us harm. Over the years I've seen countless people whose ideas about wellness had morphed into a sneaky form of disordered eating that was taking over their lives, and I was in that exact same boat myself ten to fifteen years ago. And that level of concern with health and wellness is anything but health-promoting.

To understand this new manifestation of diet culture and why it's so dangerous, we have to look at how and why the national conversation about food shifted around the turn of the millennium. It all started with a growing concern about the food industry.

Food Activism and Diet Culture

The food-activist movement that emerged in the early 2000s certainly doesn't appear on the surface to be an extension of diet culture. One of its primary aims was to make people aware of the political and economic forces shaping our food system, and to increase access to foods produced in a sustainable way with a minimal toll on the environment. Food activism is in many ways the intellectual descendant of the health-food movement that began in the 1960s and '70s. Unfortunately, though, the twenty-first-century brand of food activism was also intertwined from the start with the concept of the "obesity epidemic," and through that connection it reinforced weight stigma and continues to uphold the diet-culture principle that smaller bodies are both healthier and more morally correct.

The 2001 bestseller *Fast Food Nation* was this movement's first major text. Author Eric Schlosser did some impressive investigative journalism to build the case that the fast-food industry had shaped the American landscape and deepened income inequality, and that we need to change the system in order to correct these injustices. Unfortunately, Schlosser also unquestioningly embraced one of the modern tenets of diet culture, arguing that the fast-food industry had made this country into not just a nation of "obese" people but an "empire of fat." "The obesity epidemic that began in the United States during the 1970s is now spreading to the rest of the world, with fast food as one of its vectors," Schlosser wrote ominously.[6] Fast food was infecting the world with the "disease" of fatness. For devotees of the food-activist movement, the connection between fast food and so-called "obesity" may seem self-evident now, but that's largely because of the far-reaching influence of Schlosser's book and other early food-activist works. Citing the Dietz-Mokdad research as well as dozens of news articles about the ostensible epidemic, Schlosser framed "obesity" as a public-health crisis—and blamed the fast-food industry for its spread. In my view, this argument is deeply flawed for a number of reasons. For one thing, as we'll discuss shortly, arguments about how the food industry or the "standard American diet" is purportedly creating an "obesity epidemic" are intertwined with racist and classist beliefs. For another, no type of food is inherently good or bad, as you'll see in Chapter 9. And that's to say nothing of the fact that pointing fingers at the food industry conveniently deflects attention from diet culture, which deserves a lot more scrutiny than it gets in the food-activist movement.

Whereas the alleged "obesity epidemic" is a fabrication, any true uptick in the national average BMI over the years tracks nicely with the continued growth of the diet industry and diet culture in general—including the emergence of public-health initiatives aimed at changing the food environment so that people will cut their consumption of fast food and other high-calorie options.[7] Clearly these initiatives aren't having the intended effect. Steady pressure on people to shrink their bodies for the last century and a half hasn't resulted in any lasting reduction in people's weights, and we know from the research that intentional weight loss often makes people heavier in the long run. Again, there's nothing wrong with being in a larger body—it's our society's *beliefs* about larger bodies that cause the real problems—but if the average body size in the Westernized world is increasing, it may have less to do with the much-maligned "Western diet" than with diet *culture*, a uniquely Western export. We don't have an "obesity epidemic," but we sure as hell do have a diet-culture epidemic.

Fast Food Nation was the first in a steady stream of food-activist books and films that came out in the early 2000s, all with variations on the same theme. In 2002 nutrition-policy expert Marion Nestle published *Food Politics*, a scholarly text on the role of the food industry in shaping our nutrition and health, which galvanized a generation of food writers and health professionals (myself included). "As a population, Americans are eating more animal-based foods—and more food in general—to the point where half of us are overweight, even our children are obese, and diseases related to diet are leading causes of death and disability," Nestle wrote in the book's preface.[8] She builds her argument against the food industry on the assumptions that larger body size equals poor health, and that overeating or eating particular types of food is the cause of larger body size— suppositions that are based on diet-culture beliefs rather than on scientific fact.

The film *Super Size Me* made a bit of a splash in 2004, but the food movement truly hit the mainstream with journalist Michael Pollan's bestselling book *The Omnivore's Dilemma* in 2006. Echoing Schlosser's words, Pollan called America "a republic of fat" created by processed food and government-subsidized, large-scale agriculture. "When food is abundant and cheap, people will eat more of it and get fat," Pollan wrote confidently, continuing in diet culture's long tradition of demonizing fatness and attributing weight gain to a combination of food-industry greed and poor individual decision-making.[9] He argued that we need to change the food system by buying our ingredients from local, small-scale, sustainable farmers and artisans, and cooking from scratch instead of relying on processed food.

Although that argument has been criticized for being elitist and out of touch with the financial realities of millions of people who can't afford to eat that way, Pollan's book was tremendously popular and persuasive, not to mention well written. It was chosen as one of the *New York Times Book Review*'s ten best books of 2006; five years later *Time* magazine named it one of the "100 best and most influential" books written in English since the magazine's founding in 1923. *The Omnivore's Dilemma* helped inspire an explosion of farm-to-table cuisine in the mid- to late 2000s, when suddenly it seemed like every chef and their mom was extolling the virtues of knowing your farmer. As the *Time* review put it, "One has to wonder if Michelle Obama would have chosen to plant a White House garden had it not been for Pollan and the huge influence he's had on chefs, consumers and the culture of American eating."

It's hard for me to talk about this period in the evolution of diet culture without also mentioning my own history. When I was a twenty-two-year-old newbie journalist struggling in my own relationship with food and searching for a beat to call my own, reading *Fast Food Nation* and *Food Politics* helped change the course of my career—and fanned the flames of my eating disorder. Those books helped drive my choice to focus on food politics in my work as a writer and editor. Later, in my mid-twenties, *The Omnivore's Dilemma* took me even deeper into the food-activist movement, giving my diet-addled brain new things to fixate on (namely eating local and avoiding "industrial" foods at all costs). At that time I could see no downsides to this way of eating and living; these authors were heroes to me, role models of how to build a career as a food writer with an activist streak.

In 2007 I interviewed Pollan for a Q&A on the *Gourmet* website, and several years later I applied for the food-and-farming journalism fellowship he founded at my alma mater, UC Berkeley (I didn't get it, which proved to be for the best). I chose NYU for graduate school primarily because I wanted to study with *Food Politics* author Nestle. I took her class on food politics and even got some advice from her on career issues. She and Pollan both struck me as kind, smart people who want to do good in the world. And frankly, I do still occasionally enjoy eating in the ways they advocate, such as shopping at farmers' markets and cooking elaborate meals from scratch. But as I healed my own relationship with food and delved into the field of disordered eating and the history of diet culture, I came to understand just how much unintentional harm their work—and the food-activist movement in general—has caused.

This harm is particularly clear in Pollan's next book, *In Defense of Food,* published in 2008. It begins with what has become one of the most famous passages in modern food writing: "Eat food. Not too much. Mostly plants."[10] That's Pollan's food-activist advice for how to approach nourishment; he inveighs against "nutritionism," the practice of looking at food in terms of its component nutrients, which had emerged with the rise of nutrition science and the discovery of vitamins in the early 1900s. Pollan rightly points out that nutritionism takes us away from the true beauty and pleasure of food and does little to support our health, but he also sets up a moral hierarchy of food that places so-called "real" foods (such as locally grown vegetables and pasture-raised meat) at the top and anything "processed" or mass-produced at the bottom. That famous passage became a yardstick for people to measure their eating against—and to beat themselves with when they didn't measure up.

Now, in addition to worrying about calories, fat, or carbs (because it's not like those concerns went away), you had to worry about whether the food you ate was "real" enough, whether your portions were the "right" size or "too much," and whether you had "enough" plants on your plate. You also still had to worry about "obesity," which Pollan refers to as a disease and an epidemic throughout the book. Indeed, as social-sciences professor Julie Guthman writes, "Pollan, more than any other food writer, has become carried away with linking growing girth to the US food system."[11]

Pollan sharpened the edges of the yardstick even more with his 2009 book, *Food Rules: An Eater's Manual,* a concise follow-up to *In Defense of Food* that was meant to give more concrete guidance and, well, rules about what to eat or avoid.[12] But for Americans, given all that we've been through in our national relationship with food and our bodies—well over a century's worth of weight stigma, diet-industry pressure, and body shame—food rules are inextricably bound up with diet culture. And because we live in diet culture, we're all conditioned to *want* rules about food—which is likely why Pollan's publisher signed him up to write the book, and why his audience was receptive to it. As well-intentioned as I'm sure Pollan was in writing it, there's no way that food rules could be viewed as anything other than a diet by most readers—even if those rules were framed as a "lifestyle change" or "getting healthy." In Western society in the twenty-first century, where there are rules about what to eat, there's diet culture.

That's the thing about the food-activist movement: it misses a critical piece of the story about food in our culture. For all their attunement to the impact of industry pressure on our food system and our health, food activists left a huge stone unturned by overlooking the influence of the pharmaceutical and weight-loss industries on the fabrication of the "obesity epidemic." By introducing the notion that our food system contributes to this so-called epidemic, these activists unwittingly allied themselves with diet culture. Because food-activist arguments generally focus not on cutting calories or fat but on food politics, public health, and eating (often delicious) locally produced food, however, the alliance with diet culture might not be obvious at first glance.

The movement's anti-food-industry sentiment has distracted people from the fact that by and large, food activists have built their case for changing the food system on a foundation of weight stigma, which directly benefits the weight-loss industry and harms everyday people, particularly those in larger bodies. There are other distractions, too: Pollan, Nestle, and other prominent food activists are public intellectuals rather than, say, doctors, "wellness influencers," or personal trainers, which makes their books seem more like cultural touchstones than diet books—even though in many ways the latter is exactly what they are. Moreover, food activism ignores the fact that the roots of our cultural preference for thinness and weight loss are planted in the racist hierarchy of bodies created by nineteenth-century evolutionary biologists. The food movement considers itself socially progressive, yet it unintentionally upholds an outmoded, racist, oppressive view of bodies by accepting and repeating "obesity epidemic" rhetoric and blaming particular foods for supposedly making people fat.

Indeed, arguments about how our food system is ostensibly

creating an "obesity epidemic" are deeply intertwined with racism. The food movement views fatness in what Saguy calls a sociocultural frame, blaming larger body size on a "toxic food environment" that includes easy access to "fattening" food and lack of access to "healthy" food.[13] Her research has found that the sociocultural frame gets applied disproportionately to people of color, especially black and Latinx folks, and that it targets such cultural practices as the food choices of these groups. Even when the supposed problem is construed in terms of society rather than individuals, the supposed solutions are still all about individual responsibility—teaching people how to navigate the food environment in order to make "better choices," and assuming that cultural culinary practices are at fault. This emphasis on individual choices includes teaching people of color to give up culturally important foods in favor of "healthier" ones as defined by the dominant (aka white) culture.

In this way, Guthman points out, the food movement's efforts to get people to eat "better" has a lot in common with early colonial efforts to convert native and indigenous peoples to a European way of eating.[14] Just as Europeans saw themselves as teaching other groups how to do food, religion, and everyday life in the "correct" way, the food-activist movement is all about instructing low-income groups and people of color how to "make the right choices" about what they eat—which generally means forgoing cheaper and more convenient options in favor of "whole" foods that cost more money and require more labor to prepare.

Those foods might appeal to the white elites who make up the overwhelming majority of the food movement, but they're certainly not universally desired. Food-activist programs therefore generally contain an educational component that's all about instructing less-privileged groups in matters of culinary taste—which harks back to various efforts by white, privileged people throughout history to "civilize" people of color. The food movement also implies that if you eat what it deems to be the right foods, you'll avoid "obesity" and end up thin, just like Pollan, Nestle, and other (overwhelmingly white) food-activist leaders. In this way the food-activist movement upholds white culture's preference for thinness by equating it with the picture of health, and defines "real food" as the type preferred by white elites.

I understood none of this when I myself was one of those privileged white people in the food-activist movement. But several years later, as I began working with clients with eating disorders, I started waking up to just how problematic food activism was. I saw people who ran themselves ragged trying to eat in the ways that Pollan, Nestle, and their ilk recommended. It took me back to my own disordered-eating days, when I would agonize for hours over whether to buy the nonorganic local kale or the organic bunch that had been shipped cross-country, the "processed" gluten-free granola bar or the "small-batch" bar with gluten, the grass-fed whole milk from the farmers' market or the "industrial" vegan milk from the grocery store. Getting caught up in these kinds of concerns, I realized, was causing my clients tremendous pain and robbing them of untold time and mental energy, just as it had for me. And I started to see how telling people they "should" be eating "whole, minimally processed" foods didn't differ much from telling them they "should" be eating low-fat, low-carb, or low-calorie foods. It was all part of the larger system of policing what people ate under the guise of improving their health—and it was harming all of us.

From Gluten Hysteria to Clean Eating

At the end of the twentieth century, the general public had never even heard of gluten. A few years later, gluten-free diets were a global phenomenon—in part thanks to a doctor named Alessio Fasano, who never set out to create a diet-culture trend. Now the director of the Center for Celiac Research and Treatment at Massachusetts General Hospital, Fasano started out as a pediatric gastroenterologist in Naples, Italy, where he saw many cases of celiac disease. The disease is characterized by an inability to digest gluten—a protein found in wheat, rye, and barley—and was well-known in Europe in the 1980s and 1990s. But when Fasano moved to the United States in 1993, he was surprised to hear American researchers and physicians call celiac disease extraordinarily rare in their country. *That can't be right,* thought Fasano, so he started to study the prevalence of the disease in the U.S.

In one of his best-known studies, Fasano and a team of researchers examined atypical and "silent" manifestations of celiac disease in a way that no American scientists had before. Ultimately, they found that 0.75 percent of the more than 4,100 "not-at-risk" subjects in his study actually had the disease—a far greater percentage than anyone had previously thought, even though it was still less than 1 percent.[15] The results of this research were published in 2003 in the journal *Archives of Internal Medicine,* sparking a wave of scientific interest in celiac disease. Fasano's research also had drawn more attention to gluten in general, inspiring some American scientists to start looking for links between gluten and health problems other than celiac disease.

It wasn't just scientists, though; the world of complementary and alternative medicine (CAM) was keenly interested in gluten around the turn of the millennium as well, and CAM proponents were some of the earliest adopters of the gluten-free trend. And whereas the newfound attention to celiac was a blessing to those with this condition, the tsunami of interest in gluten itself would wind up problematic at best. This isn't to say that all forms of CAM are inherently problematic; there are some wonderful naturopathic and integrative physicians out there who understand the problems with diet culture and the current wellness trend and are doing innovative work to help people recover from disordered eating. Unfortunately, that's not the majority of the CAM world. Like Western medical practitioners, most CAM providers are caught up in diet culture, and many have perpetuated (and indeed helped create) the sneaky new form of diet culture that pretends to be all about wellness. It's these segments of the CAM world I'm discussing here.

I myself became obsessed with gluten sometime in late 2003—just as I was getting into the food-activist movement—when a family friend who was into alternative medicine suggested that my missing periods, fatigue, digestive troubles, and "brain fog" could perhaps be fixed by going gluten-free. This was during a time when I was jumping from doctor to doctor trying to get a diagnosis for what were simply complications of my disordered eating and overexercise, but no one knew that then. Many doctors didn't ask me about my eating or physical activity, and the ones who did ask saw nothing wrong with what I was doing. Because my BMI was in the so-called "normal" range as opposed to "underweight," they deemed my rigid habits "healthy." So instead of getting help for my disordered eating, I started researching gluten and tumbled headlong into message boards filled with people blaming the wheat-derived protein for conditions such as autism, schizophrenia, and general malaise, with no good evidence to support their claims. That lack of evidence didn't bother me at the time, though. I was looking for something—anything—to explain my health problems, and gluten became an easy scapegoat.

I want to be clear: For people with actual celiac disease or wheat allergy, a gluten-free or wheat-free menu is a medical necessity, and decades of solid science back that up. For people without those conditions, though, there's no good evidence that cutting out wheat or gluten brings any benefit. The practice of going gluten-free to "heal the gut" can in fact mask disordered eating—a much more likely cause of digestive troubles than gluten, given that as many as *98 percent* of people with eating disorders have gastrointestinal disorders,[16] and that up to 44 percent of general patients seeking help for gastrointestinal problems have disordered-eating behaviors.[17] Moreover, the tests that some health practitioners use to diagnose so-called gluten sensitivity and other "food intolerances"—including hair analysis, applied kinesiology, and blood tests from labs that yield long, color-coded lists of foods to avoid—lack scientific validity.[18] Their results are no better at predicting food sensitivities than chance, so you'd be better off asking a Magic 8 Ball whether you were intolerant to gluten; at least it wouldn't charge you hundreds of dollars out of pocket. (Speaking of which, those tests aren't covered by insurance because they're so bogus that insurance companies wouldn't touch them with a ten-foot pole. They don't meet the criteria for evidence-based medicine.)

None of this stopped the media (including yours truly) from fanning the flames of the emerging gluten-free trend. From 2005 to 2008 I wrote several articles about gluten, trying to follow ever-stricter versions of the gluten-free diet along the way. Never mind that I had tested negative for celiac disease numerous times by that point, or that I still wasn't entirely sure whether cutting out gluten was making me feel any better (even though I told everyone that it was, to help justify my continued food restriction). I got great feedback on those articles from my editors, and persuaded a number of people I knew to try going gluten-free. Soon fellow journalists started covering all the celebrities who were jumping aboard the trend: Oprah and Gwyneth Paltrow were doing gluten-free cleanses, and Jenny McCarthy had put her son on the diet. In 2009, Elisabeth Hasselbeck (then cohost of *The View*) released a bestselling book called *The G-Free Diet,* in which she claimed that going gluten-free could help you heal myriad symptoms and, of course, lose weight. (Like every other diet under the sun, the gluten-free diet has *not* been shown to produce lasting weight loss.)

More books soon followed, including *Wheat Belly* in 2011 and *Grain Brain* in 2013, two bestsellers that demonized gluten and grains for supposedly causing weight gain, cognitive decline, and a host of other conditions—all based on science that I would characterize as woefully inadequate, at best. Many medical experts and media outlets have called out these books for dispensing pseudoscience and unsubstantiated quackery.[19] Yet food manufacturers rushed into the new niche, and the U.S. market for gluten-free foods grew from $580 million in 2004 to $1.85 billion in 2018, with the global market following suit.

In the early 2000s, food activism and the gluten-free fad had cross-pollinated to create what would become one of the most popular manifestations of modern diet culture: "clean eating." Combining the fetishization of "real food" with the demonization of gluten and other grains, the concept of clean eating had its origins in alternative medicine and made its way into the bodybuilding world; it was then popularized by bodybuilder and bikini competitor Tosca Reno in her 2005 book, *The Eat-Clean Diet.* Her version of clean eating was a low-calorie diet with a twist: it encouraged people to eat "whole foods" and to avoid artificial ingredients, preservatives, sugar, and anything "processed" (in addition to controlling calories and portion size, like pretty much all diets). Lots of smoothies were involved. In 2008 Reno cofounded *Clean Eating* magazine with her husband, Robert Kennedy (a British-born fitness-media publisher, no relation to the American political dynasty), and a few years later she wrote a follow-up diet book that further spread the gospel of clean eating. When Facebook acquired Instagram in 2012, the latter's millions of new users made #cleaneating a viral trend. With its photogenic foods such as green juices and colorful salads—and eventually the now-ubiquitous smoothie bowl—clean eating was poised for Instagram stardom.

Clean eating has no single official definition, making it even harder to pin down than other sneaky forms of diet culture. It's defined variously as eating only organic, sustainable, "whole" foods and avoiding anything "processed"—which, taken to the extreme, can leave you with a woefully limited menu, because everything we eat is processed to a degree. Some people interpret "clean" to mean eating only vegetarian or vegan; others take it even further and consider only *raw* vegan foods to be clean. Many definitions include an avoidance of gluten, and some make all grains and starches off-limits.

What all the definitions have in common is a fixation on dietary purity and categorizing food in terms of virtue and vice: *clean* vs. *dirty, real* vs. *fake, whole* vs. *processed,* and *pure* vs. *contaminated.* Harking back to Sylvester Graham and his austere Grahamite diet, clean eating is wrapped up in morality—the idea that right-thinking, upstanding people "eat clean," and if you slip up, you need to "detox" to bring yourself back to purity. Clean eating is also bound up in the "it's-not-a-diet-it's-a-lifestyle-change" rhetoric that characterizes diet culture in the new millennium. The trend's eponymous magazine puts it this way: "*Clean Eating* is not a diet; it's real food for a healthy, happy life."[20]

Looking at clean eating with an awareness of diet culture, though, we can see that it is *definitely* a diet—just by another name. Though in some cases overt mentions of weight loss have been dropped from the discourse about clean eating, it's obvious from early iterations such as Reno's books that weight loss was the point from the start. Now the weight-stigmatizing language tends to be subtler, more coded: "These waffles will get you energized without having you feel weighed down," writes clean-eating blogger and cookbook author Carina Wolff. "If you eat garbage, your body will show it," cautions clean-eating blog *The Gracious Pantry.* "Love what you eat and look and feel like the best version of yourself," say self-styled nutrition gurus and clean-eating queens Jasmine and Melissa Hemsley.

Of course, there are plenty of overtly diet-y manifestations of clean eating as well: JJ Smith, a nutritionist and author of multiple books about green-smoothie cleanses, touts clean eating as part of her "breakthrough permanent weight loss solution" (when in reality no diet can create permanent weight loss for the overwhelming majority of people, as we'll discuss in Chapter 3); the authors of the book *Clean Cuisine* promise "hunger-free weight loss" (nope, not a thing); and Tosca Reno's Eat-Clean Diet® brand is still hawking weight loss and still going strong, now with a registered trademark and a host of new cleanses and programs (which, like all diets, are backed up by NO sound scientific evidence of long-term "success"). It's likewise common for clean-eating Instagrammers to add hashtags such as #weightlossjourney, #lowcarb, and #diet to their posts, belying any claims that clean eating is not about weight or dieting.

There's also the issue of moralizing about different styles of eating, a trait of diet culture that's become more and more prominent over the years. Calling a particular way of eating "clean" automatically labels anything else unclean or dirty. It makes people afraid they'll become riddled with "toxins" and disease if they eat the "wrong" thing. And it creates an imagined moral hierarchy in which people who "eat clean" are viewed (or view themselves) as morally superior to those who don't (and feel incredibly guilty if they deviate from the supposedly correct diet). In that sense, clean eating has echoes of religious dietary laws.

As explained by Alan Levinovitz, a religious-studies professor at James Madison University and author of *The Gluten Lie: And Other Myths About What You Eat,* many people in this day and age treat diets like religions—even in the secular world. "Modern dietary practices conceal quasi-religious rituals under the language of science," he says. "In the same way that your religion becomes your identity, your dietary practices and rituals and your beliefs about which foods are clean and unclean become who you are." Diets provide a system of beliefs to organize behavior, a way of identifying yourself (whether as a "clean eater" or an adherent of some other type of diet) and a community of others who share those beliefs.

There's nothing wrong with those things in and of themselves—we all need a value system, an identity, and a community. The problem is that in the case of clean eating and other modern manifestations of diet culture, the belief system often takes over your life and prevents you from developing your own identity and values *outside* food and eating. It shrinks your life by making you more and more fixated on food and exercise, at the expense of other things you truly care about. Clean eating isn't alone in that. With *all* forms of diet culture, the message is that you can't trust yourself and that you have to follow its rules in order to be saved—and the longer and harder you try to adhere to it, the more it crowds out other areas of your life.

Moreover, clean eating is particularly conducive to the notion that if you aren't seeing any benefits, it's because you aren't eating clean *enough*. "There's a very poisonous kind of religious belief in which whenever you're failing or whenever you're unhappy it's because you're not being holy enough," Levinovitz says. "And so you pray more, you sacrifice more, you self-flagellate more, and that can be an endless cycle where you feel worse and worse." In the case of clean eating and other modern dietary practices, people start cutting out foods and pursuing dietary "purity," only to feel worse because now they're isolating themselves from friends and cutting off access to pleasurable foods. Instead of realizing that the problem lies with the diet, however, they believe that the solution is to diet *harder* and eliminate *more* foods, because they blame themselves for "doing it wrong" rather than blaming the diet for not working. When people get into that cycle, they can end up with a severely limited menu that harms their health—ironic, given that health is the supposed point of the diet in the first place.

Orthorexia and the Modern Condition

In the mid-1990s, integrative-medicine physician Steven Bratman observed something troubling in his practice. Many of his patients were coming in as fairly well-adjusted people who wanted help dealing with relatively minor health issues such as eczema or asthma. But as they followed his advice to eliminate certain foods to help their conditions, these patients became obsessed with food and nutrition—to the detriment of their lives. They stopped going out much, if at all, and when they did leave the house they traveled with containers full of their own food. They isolated themselves from friends and family. They even ended relationships with people who were otherwise wonderful but did not fit into their extreme ways of eating.

Bratman estimates that this food-obsessive behavior showed up in as many as half of his patients. He began to realize that the "food as medicine" prescription could be worse than whatever ailment these patients were trying to manage. "I eventually came to regard food allergy treatment as the equivalent of a dangerous medication, one that should be prescribed only sparingly," he later wrote.[21]

In an effort to help these patients recognize and recover from their food fixations, Bratman coined a medical-sounding term to "diagnose" them: *orthorexia nervosa,* which translates roughly as "obsession with 'correct' eating." Bratman meant it as a slightly tongue-in-cheek way of telling his patients they had a problem, and it worked: "The word turned expectations upside down and opened a pathway to further discussion," he explains. In the late 1990s and early 2000s, after Bratman published articles and eventually a book about the phenomenon, the medical community began to recognize orthorexia as a very real form of disordered eating—one that fixates on the supposed health and purity of food as opposed to its calorie content.

The concept of orthorexia also struck a chord with the general public: when *Cosmopolitan* published a story about this newly discovered form of disordered eating, the writer told Bratman that the article got a bigger reaction than any of her food columns. Orthorexia came even further into mainstream consciousness in 2014, when blogger Jordan Younger—then known as The Blonde Vegan—announced to her massive audience that she was suffering from the condition and needed to start breaking her dietary restrictions in order to recover. Major media outlets such as *Good Morning America,* the *Wall Street Journal,* and *Nightline* reported on Younger's situation, which made for a compelling news story partly because she had such a huge following and partly because she was receiving death threats from angry members of her audience for daring to step away from the restrictive-eating practices that she'd championed—which included not just eschewing animal products but also being gluten-free, eating only raw foods, and doing lots of cleanses. (Younger subsequently rebranded herself as The Balanced Blonde, speaking out about orthorexia recovery and moving away from extreme wellness pursuits for a few years. As of early 2019, however, she had reverted to promoting restrictive-eating behaviors and selling cleanses.)

It turns out that people are particularly susceptible to orthorexia when they start following elimination diets (cutting out a wide variety of foods in an effort to pinpoint any sensitivities) and other restrictive or extreme dietary theories, especially ones that moralize about food. Clean eating—especially #cleaneating on Instagram—definitely falls into that camp: a 2017 study showed that higher Instagram use was associated with a greater likelihood of having orthorexia (an effect not seen with any other social-media channel), and nearly *half* of the Instagram users surveyed met criteria for orthorexia.[22] But as Bratman notes, orthorexia can happen with any dietary theory. Whereas the most restrictive and pseudoscientific diets are the riskiest, people can develop orthorexia by following even governmental dietary guidelines in an extreme way.

Orthorexia is a serious subject of study in the eating-disorder field today, though it's still a long way from inclusion in the *Diagnostic and Statistical Manual of Mental Disorders,* the bible of "official" mental-health diagnoses. As to whether orthorexia *should* be an official diagnosis, scientific opinion is mixed. Even Bratman has some reservations, primarily because orthorexia has much in common with existing eating disorders: "Orthorexia is beginning to seem to me more like a variation of anorexia rather than an independent condition," he says. " 'Healthy' and 'low calorie' have begun to converge in the popular mind, and it is hard to find people with orthorexia who aren't also concerned about body weight." He sees shifting cultural norms as the main reason why these two variations of disordered eating have started to seem so similar. "In my initial observations in the 1990s," wrote Bratman in 2017, "orthorexia arose primarily in alternative-medicine subcultures where specific healthy food diets are espoused. Subsequently, interest in healthy eating has pervaded popular culture."[23]

Indeed, in a way that was inconceivable in the 1990s, people now constantly share their opinions about whatever they consider to be "healthy" food on blogs and social media, and food companies market their products as "healthy" rather than low-calorie. The invention of the "obesity epidemic" also served to mainstream the conflation of weight and health, which means the pursuit of a thin body and the pursuit of a healthy body are now generally seen as one and the same. In my clinical practice, all the clients I've treated for orthorexia have worried that their recovery efforts would make them gain weight, and all those I've treated for anorexia expressed concern that pursuing recovery was making them less healthy.

In the end, I'm not sure it matters if orthorexia is labeled as its own eating disorder or part of another one. In fact, distinguishing eating disorders as a category separate from the "normal" pathology of dieting serves merely to entrench diet culture further. Drawing that distinction can distract us from the fact that all eating problems—whether diagnosed or not—are part of the same larger system. Imagine anorexia, binge-eating disorder, and all other clinical eating-disorder diagnoses as different species of redwoods, while dieting and subclinical disordered eating are Douglas firs: they're all part of the same massive woodland, and often we lose sight of the forest for the trees.

Sure, the distinctions among different types of trees matter to botanists, just as the distinctions among various eating disorders and subclinical eating pathologies matter to scientific researchers and the creators of diagnostic tools. But what the average person really cares about is that there are big wild woods out there; traipse through them without the right gear and we might get lost and die. Or in the case of diet culture, there's a massive system of pathological eating behaviors and body-image concerns out there; go into it unaware and we're almost certain to get our lives stolen—at least in the figurative sense, if not worse.

Understanding and learning how to navigate this system is essential for our survival. The tree analogy breaks down a bit when it comes to the idea of dismantling diet culture: I would never advocate destroying a forest, but there's a good argument to be made for burning diet culture to the ground. And if we truly want to support people's well-being, that's what we need to do. (As you'll learn in Part II, there are plenty of ways to care for your health that don't involve diet culture's rules, restrictions, or moralistic ideas about food and bodies.)

By the way, the diet-culture forest eventually swallows up even those forms of disordered eating that develop in response to individual factors such as trauma, self-esteem issues, and other life circumstances. Disordered-eating behaviors don't exist in a vacuum. If you start eating to soothe yourself after experiencing trauma, for example, you're not doing that in a culture of "Do what you gotta do to get through the day, and also let me help you process your trauma." No, you're doing it in a culture of "OMG YOU'RE EATING SO MUCH, YOU'RE GONNA GAIN

WEIGHT AND THAT'S ABSOLUTELY UNACCEPTABLE—
YOU NEED TO LOSE WEIGHT, STAT! (And PS, *trauma*? What
are you even talking about? Just suck it up and move on!)"

So even when people start eating to self-soothe, without any
connection to weight or body image, they eventually end up
absorbing our culture's toxic beliefs about food and bodies. In
our society at this moment in history, it's basically impossible *not*
to fall into diet culture's clutches at some point. As you'll see in
later chapters, however, it *is* possible to extricate yourself and
move beyond it.

The Wellness Diet

Clean eating, Whole30, Paleo, intermittent fasting, detoxing...
since the turn of the millennium, diet culture has become such
a shape-shifter that it's hard to keep up with all its new manifestations. From the time I write these words to the moment you
read them, a whole new crop of trendy diets will undoubtedly
come on the market. But with very few exceptions, modern-day
diets have one thing in common: They claim not to be diets.
They say they're about health and wellness, not dieting.

Even when they have the word *diet* in their name, they're
quick to assure you that they're not diets per se. (Most of them
opt for terms such as *protocol, reset, reboot, cleanse, detox, program,
template, eating plan,* or *lifestyle* instead.) Whatever they call themselves, though, know this: they're all part of the sneaky, modern
guise of diet culture that's supposedly about wellness but is actually about *performing* a rarefied, perfectionistic, discriminatory
idea of what health is supposed to look like. I refer to diets like
these collectively as the Wellness Diet, to highlight the fact that
they are diets cloaking themselves as wellness.

These sneaky diets like to pretend they're unique—*totally
different* from every other "protocol," "plan," or "lifestyle" out there.

But the truth is they're all remarkably similar; they're all born from the same diet culture that gave us calorie counting, Grahamites, and the Banting diet more than a century ago, and that now shows up in more covert forms such as the "obesity epidemic," food activism, and the obsession with cutting out gluten and other maligned foods. Just like the overt diets of decades past, the Wellness Diet is about eating the supposedly "right" things and removing the supposedly "wrong" ones, all in a bid to attain a state of moral and bodily "correctness" (which of course includes thinness).

The argument that "It's about health, not dieting!" is in fact central to diet culture's business model in this day and age. Consider these words from a 2017 report by Marketdata, an independent market-research publisher that also offers consulting and strategic planning to the diet industry: "'Diet' has become a four-letter word in the minds of many consumers. 'Healthy' eating has replaced 'dieting.'"[24] The diet industry, in other words, knows exactly what it's doing when it frames its interventions as "lifestyle changes" and "healthy hacks" rather than diets. Indeed, it *has* to do this in order to survive: "Any weight loss company that continues to focus most of their efforts on Baby Boomers is sure to wither and die," the Marketdata report continues. "Many Millennials today view Weight Watchers and Jenny Craig as your mother's (or grandmother's) weight loss program. This will be the challenge—to stay relevant and cultivate this future generation of dieters."

Predictably, since that report was published Weight Watchers changed its name to "WW" in an effort to rebrand itself as a "health and wellness" company that goes beyond, well, weight watching. The 2018 name change came with a new tagline— "Wellness That Works"—and a new effort to appeal to people who want to "get healthy" without necessarily focusing on weight loss or dieting. "This idea of going from weight to wellness is more sustainable to people because we're giving them more than just a short-term solution," WW president and CEO Mindy Grossman told the *Today* show the day of the rebranding announcement. In so doing, she came surprisingly close to admitting something that has been common knowledge in the scientific community since the 1960s: intentional weight loss is not sustainable long-term. Or, as Grossman put it in numerous interviews leading up to the announcement, "healthy is the new skinny." Her phrasing helps clarify that the rebrand caters to people's ongoing desire for thinness while pretending to be about the seemingly more laudable goal of health. And not just any kind of health, but a certain *perception* of health that's trendy right now. "[Millennials'] weight loss efforts are likely to focus on clean eating, exercise, convenience, and avoiding artificial sweeteners and highly processed foods," Marketdata president John LaRosa wrote in 2018.[25]

So when you see traditional diet companies rebranding them-selves in ways that seem hip and modern, it's not because they care about what's good for people's health—it's because they're trying to stay afloat by appealing to a younger generation, and they see wellness messaging as the way to do that. To capture the lucrative millennial market, diet companies have to make prod-ucts and services that align with the trend of "It's not about weight, it's about wellness." That includes offerings such as meal-kit-delivery services, recipe apps, diet books, protein powders, and meal-replacement bars built around "whole foods" and "clean eating." Sure enough, in early 2019 WW retooled its food-and-beverage products to remove all artificial sweeteners, flavors, col-ors, and preservatives—a move that affected 70 percent of those products, but that WW believes will boost sales.[26] Wellness is big business for the diet industry.

The Wellness Diet isn't just about weight, but thinness is an essential part of its supposed picture of health. So are youth, physical ability, wealth, and whiteness—or at least Eurocentric features, if you're not white. The thin (or "lean," as the fitness community likes to say), young, able-bodied, and mostly white bodies of wellness "influencers" are held up as paragons of health. The implication is that if you eat and exercise like them—which involves a lot of smoothie bowls, green juices, and expensive fitness classes—you'll end up looking like them. While they may be somewhat less emaciated and more muscular than the waiflike models of the 1990s, they still have very thin bodies that the vast majority of the population cannot attain. (The same goes for their incessantly Instagrammed eating and exercise habits, which can consume an entire paycheck faster than you can say "chia seeds.")

In that sense, wellness influencers are the Gibson Girls of the twenty-first century—supposedly liberating images of beauty and vitality that are actually oppressive. Just as the Gibson Girl *seemed* more liberated than the Victorian beauty ideal, proponents of the Wellness Diet might at first appear less bound by the strictures of diet culture. They don't seem to be starving themselves, after all; as the Hemsley sisters write, "We don't believe in depriving ourselves of treats and comfort foods, we just make them using whole ingredients and unrefined, natural sweeteners."[27] Of course, constantly substituting Wellness Diet–approved ingredients for traditional ones *is* a form of deprivation, and a "slipup" with "processed" or "refined" foods usually requires atonement in the form of a cleanse or "reset."

Among other diet-culture mainstays of the Wellness Diet: characterizing certain foods as "bad," "toxic," or "junk" but others as "good," "real," or "pure"; engaging in all kinds of disordered behaviors to trick your body into eating less; and equating weight with health, only in subtler language that talks about "reaching your ideal weight" and "getting a better body" as merely a few of the program's *many* benefits. These days the Wellness Diet is even co-opting intuitive eating—the explicitly anti-diet approach to food that many of my colleagues and I use to help people break free of diet culture and get back in touch with their bodies' instincts about what, when, and how much to eat—and recasting it as a surefire path to weight loss, aka another diet. (Which it most certainly is not, as we'll discuss.) Just as the literal corset of the Victorian era was replaced by the "inner corset" of self-denial around the turn of the twentieth century, so the overt dieting of the twentieth century has been replaced by the Wellness Diet in the twenty-first.

Many Wellness Diet proponents admit to having struggled with body-image issues and a troubled relationship with food in the past, and now they frame their "protocol" or "reset" as a path to peace with food—not recognizing that they've simply traded in one form of disordered eating for another. Melissa Hartwig Urban of Whole30, Rachel Mansfield of the *RachLMansfield* food blog, and Jasmine Hemsley of the Hemsley sisters are just a few of the wellness influencers who've spoken publicly about their checkered histories with food. That these women have struggled is unsurprising, and nothing to be ashamed of—we live in diet culture, so of course they have (as have I, and in all likelihood as have you). It's the fact that they're selling their diets as the *solution* to eating issues—the path to healing and "food freedom"—that's the problem. As any good eating-disorder clinician will tell you, it's all too easy to fall into the trap of pseudo-liberation by engaging in subclinical disordered eating or chronic dieting that doesn't fit a diagnosable category or cause immediately obvious medical complications. Yet that's just as mentally distressing as any full-blown eating disorder—and sometimes even more so, given the lack of support for these less-obvious food issues.

Society looks the other way when it comes to seemingly less-severe forms of disordered eating, because diet culture has so thoroughly normalized "having food issues." So by hawking diets as the way to heal from problematic relationships with food, peddlers of the Wellness Diet keep many of their followers stuck in a pseudo-recovered place that's actually harming them. As Hartwig Urban put it in a 2018 social-media post about her eating habits, "I use the information I've learned from my dozen Whole30s and mini-resets to create the perfect, sustainable diet for me.... I play around with this, seeing how much I can 'get away with' while still looking and feeling exactly as awesome as I want to look and feel." Here she's talking about eating in a particular way in order to achieve a particular look, and sampling a bunch of diets in order to figure out the "perfect" one to follow, rather than rejecting diets (aka resets) and diet culture altogether. Hartwig Urban certainly isn't alone in thinking about food in these instrumental terms; most people do in diet culture. She's also a grown woman who's free to do whatever she wants with her body, no matter what I or anyone else has to say about it. But from my vantage point as a clinician who specializes in disordered eating, this is *not* an example of true freedom or full recovery from food and body-image issues; it's an example of dieting by another name.

Whenever I bring up the connection between so-called "wellness" and diet culture, someone always protests that what I call the Wellness Diet is really about health, not dieting. Of course I acknowledge that some people with certain health conditions (celiac disease or diabetes, for example) might benefit from making a few changes in how they eat in order to help manage those conditions. But that's not the general population. The vast majority of people don't need to eliminate any foods from their life; instead they would do better to explore the role that disordered eating might be playing in their health outcomes, as we'll discuss in Chapter 5. (Even people who are managing chronic diseases, for that matter, would benefit from letting go of disordered-eating habits.)

Meanwhile, no one needs a cleanse or a food-related detox. Unless you have an extremely rare disease that affects your liver, kidneys, or lungs, those organs already do an excellent job of removing potentially harmful substances from your body, without any intervention from you. You can in fact damage your health by engaging in detoxes and cleanses. Hell, you can even harm your health by compulsively eating fruits and vegetables. The Wellness Diet threatens your health by undermining your mental well-being—which is crucial to your overall health—and by putting you at risk of orthorexia, with all of the physical-health complications that disorder can bring.

Moreover, the way the Wellness Diet—and diet culture in general—conceives of health is bound up in *healthism:* the belief that health is a moral obligation, and that people who are "healthy" deserve more respect and resources than people who are "unhealthy" (whatever that means, and of course the definition changes to suit the person making the claim). Healthism is both a way of seeing the world that places health at the apex and a form of discriminating on the basis of health. It is both an "ism" in the sense of philosophy or ideology and an "ism" like racism or sexism. Healthism further makes health out to be exclusively a matter of individual responsibility, rather than a matter to be addressed at societal and policy levels.[28] The Wellness Diet is a fundamentally healthist point of view, framing health as the primary value in life—a duty thoughtlessly shirked by the gluten-gobbling, processed-food-devouring masses, and rectified by spending hours a day doing "meal prep," scouring restaurant menus, and hitting the spin bike.

Nutrition can certainly play a role in our overall well-being, and in the management of specific diseases. But the widespread cultural belief that "food is medicine" is problematic, to say the least. It suggests that consistently making the "right" food choices will heal or prevent all ills, and that eating certain kinds of food will inevitably harm our health. Scientific research disproves this belief by showing that people needn't cut out "processed" foods or sugar to experience good physical health, and that weight *stigma* is likely a bigger determinant of health than your actual weight or your eating

A Few Clues for Recognizing Sneaky Diet Culture

If a *wellness plan, program, protocol, reset,* or *lifestyle change* does any of the following things, you're in the presence of diet culture — no matter what it calls itself:

- Paints thinness and particular body shapes as markers of health and moral virtue
- Treats certain bodies as status symbols
- Blames BMI, weight, waist circumference, or shape for health conditions
- Talks about the "obesity epidemic" without quotation marks
- Depicts certain foods, macronutrients, or food groups as "good" and others as "bad"
- Causes anxiety and obsession about food and health
- Promotes eating smaller portions or counting/cutting calories, instead of listening to your body
- Advocates skimping on carbs or other macronutrients, and/or counting macronutrients (an important exception being if you have diabetes and need to count carbohydrates for insulin dosing—although that and other

habits. Sometimes food isn't medicine—and fixating on trying to use it as such is its own disease, known as orthorexia. In reality, there's no need to demonize certain food groups, restrict your overall food intake, or treat food as the be-all and end-all of health. In fact, putting too much emphasis on our day-to-day food choices leads not to improved health but to a preoccupation with food and panic about health. As you'll see in the next chapter, it's one of the ways diet culture steals your time—just like intentional weight loss.

forms of medical nutrition therapy can easily get twisted into diets, too)

- Automatically prescribes elimination diets for digestive concerns instead of helping heal underlying disordered eating first
- Recommends cutting out certain foods without a legitimate medical diagnosis
- Encourages detoxes and cleanses
- Tells you to wait on buying cute, comfortable clothes until you've lost weight
- Encourages you to manipulate your eating in order to shrink your body or "maintain" your size
- Promotes exercising for the purpose of weight control or body shaping
- Treats weight loss as a sign of self-actualization
- Markets weight loss as a way to "feel better" or "be more confident"
- Sets rules about what, when, how, and how much to eat (the only exception here is when you're following a meal plan for eating-disorder recovery in order to make sure you have *enough* food while you work toward restoring your body's hunger and fullness cues)

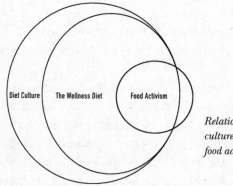

Relationship between diet and culture, the Wellness Diet, and food activism.

Diet Culture The Wellness Diet Food Activism

CHAPTER 3

How Diet Culture Steals Your Time

Anna Guest-Jelley has been on sixty-five diets in her life. That's sixty-five *distinct* diets, but some of those she tried ten times or more. She remembers that it all began at age six or seven, when her mother put her on a calorie-restricted diet at the recommendation of her pediatrician, who was concerned about where she fell on the height-weight percentiles. Her mom and a number of other family members were constantly dieting and trying to lose weight, so it felt like what she was supposed to do. By age ten, Guest-Jelley was going to Weight Watchers meetings every weekend, stepping on a scale in a room full of middle-aged adults. Instead of watching cartoons, having adventures with friends, and just being a kid, she was devoting her downtime to shrinking her body. "I was there every week weighing in, and I always felt this weird mixture of pride and shame," she says. "I would be proud on the weeks that I would lose weight, but I would always also be ashamed to be there, no matter if I lost weight or gained weight, because I was the youngest person there by far."

There would be times when she lost weight and other times when she gained it back—the classic yo-yo cycle that dieters know so well—but nothing stuck. "I left my childhood feeling like, though I was successful in school and got into a college I was excited about and had good friendships, overall my life was a failure because I couldn't lose any weight," she says. Everything else was falling into place, yet this one thing stood in the way of her feeling accomplished.

Today, as a body-acceptance advocate and founder of Curvy Yoga, an online studio and teacher-training program, Guest-Jelley sees things very differently. She never tried a sixty-sixth diet; instead, she was eventually able to make peace with her body and learn to nourish herself without dieting. But she lost untold hours of her childhood and adolescence to counting calories and points, prepping restrictive meals, and scouring menus for diet-approved options.

If you've been on even *one* diet, you probably know exactly what I'm talking about. Diet culture takes up an enormous amount of time, whether it's spent on "official" dieting programs such as the ones Guest-Jelley tried, or on more subtle things like trying on a million outfits in the morning and making yourself late for work because you "feel fat" in everything you own. Aside from the fact that *fat is not a feeling,* do you really think any of us would worry about trying to look thin in our clothes if it weren't for the primacy placed on thinness since the late 1800s? Diet culture has created this ritual that now seems like a normal part of getting dressed in the morning for countless women and trans folks, as well as for a growing number of men. And you can bet that none of us would be using the word *fat* as a synonym for *unattractive* if it weren't for diet culture.

We also sure as hell would not be exercising for the purposes of weight loss or body shaping—another way that diet culture subtly sucks away your time. Sure, it can be great for your overall well-being to move your body in ways that feel good, and some forms of movement are fun in their own right. But let's be real: shrinking and "sculpting" are major motivations for many people who exercise, and diet culture is to blame. Too many of us have gritted our teeth through workout classes and personal-training sessions we hated, all with the goal of changing our size and shape (or perhaps maintaining them, if we were already at a place that diet culture deemed "acceptable"). Think of all the ways you could've spent that time, from doing a less-intense type of movement that you actually enjoyed to working on a creative project to volunteering or doing political organizing to sitting on the couch and having some much-needed downtime.

And no, I'm not talking about sitting on the couch with your computer and diving down internet rabbit holes researching the latest diet or "lifestyle change," which is another way that diet culture usurps your time. Ragen Chastain knows that one well. Now a respected anti-diet activist (and a health coach certified by the American Council on Exercise), Chastain was once a dieter who, like so many of us, kept losing weight in the short term and inevitably regaining it in the long term, no matter how closely she stuck to whatever diet she was on at the time. She became obsessed with determining which diet would help her lose weight once and for all, and she had a helpful skill that the average diet-culture-driven internet user lacks: Chastain had studied research methods and statistical analysis in college and was well versed in how to read scientific research. So she decided to scour every weight-loss study she could find—hundreds of them in total—to find the diet with the most scientific evidence supporting it. Then she would just go on that diet, and *boom*, she'd be thin.

Except that's not what happened.

"When I got to the end of that reading, I was so completely shocked by what I found out that I went back and read them all again," Chastain says. Her astonished conclusion, after weeks of research: *no* diet has been shown to be effective over the long term for more than a tiny percentage of the population. As she puts it, "Weight loss does not meet the criteria for evidence-based medicine."

You might be as shocked to read that as Chastain was to discover it, but it's true. A robust body of evidence shows that intentional weight-loss efforts don't work; with a failure rate that many researchers agree is north of 95 percent, they're a waste of time. Let's take a look at the science and you'll see what I mean.

The Science of Diet Failure

The "more than 95 percent" statistic originated in a 1959 study by Albert Stunkard, MD, a clinician who worked in the medical weight-loss field.[1] As Stunkard later explained, "This study grew out of an attempt to resolve a paradox—the contrast between my difficulties in treating obesity and the widespread assumption that such treatment was easy and effective."[2] A psychiatrist specializing in weight loss, he was very much embedded in diet culture, even though he was also one of the first medical professionals to condemn weight-related stigma: when he passed away in 2014, his *New York Times* obituary was headlined "Dr. Albert J. Stunkard, Destigmatizer of Fat, Dies at 92." He wanted diets and weight-loss interventions to work, but instead of blaming patients for their lack of success, he suspected that the problem might be with the interventions themselves.

So Stunkard set out to find answers in the research. Poring over the scientific literature available at the time, he found hundreds of studies on weight-loss treatment that had been published since the late 1920s, but quickly realized the vast majority had serious methodological flaws. Most didn't even report the outcome of the given treatment. When they did, the results were mostly in aggregate, such as the total pounds lost by all participants in the study rather than for individual patients. Some studies failed to report on the duration of treatment; for those that did, treatment times were often laughably short. (This shady tactic is smart if you're trying to prove that a certain diet is effective, because most diets appear to work in the short term but don't lead to long-term weight loss.) Most troubling, the studies Stunkard looked at didn't account for people who dropped out of treatment—an essential factor in understanding the effectiveness of any medical intervention. If you do a study showing that 50 out of 100 participants lost weight on a particular diet, but then it turns out there were originally 200 participants enrolled and half of them dropped out, your success rate most likely just got cut in half; people tend not to drop out of diet studies that are "working" for them.

After excluding all the shoddy studies, Stunkard ended up with only eight that met high enough scientific standards to be included in his review—the best available evidence at the time. The results of those studies were disconcerting for anyone who specialized in the shrinking of bodies. They showed not only that it was quite rare for people to achieve *any* significant weight loss, but also that it was more common for people to regain most or all of the weight they'd lost than it was for them to keep it off.

Stunkard's study also included an intervention component. He partnered with dietitian Mavis McLaren-Hume at the Nutrition Clinic of New York Hospital to follow 100 patients and see how they fared with weight-loss counseling. During an initial appointment, the patients were told to restrict their calorie intake to basically the same levels seen in medical weight-loss programs today; they then had regular follow-up appointments to help them stick with the recommendations.

Two and a half years later, the researchers looked at the patients' weights. The results were even worse than what Stunkard had seen in the literature. Of the hundred participants, only twelve had been able to lose a significant amount of weight at any point during the study, and only two were maintaining that weight loss two years after treatment. The rest had either returned to their starting weight or were steadily closing in on it. What's more, thirty-nine of the patients dropped out of treatment at the Nutrition Clinic—pretty much in line with the 40 percent attrition rate we see in even the most rigorous weight-loss studies today.[3] All in all, Stunkard's intervention had a 98 percent failure rate after two years.

His study was state-of-the-art for its time, and it made a huge impact on weight-loss research. Soon after its publication, Stunkard received the American Psychiatric Association's Annual Award for Research. Over the years, the results of his study with McLaren-Hume have been quoted in countless other studies on weight, and the "more than 95 percent of weight-loss efforts fail" statistic has become a clinical adage. "I believe that this paper has been cited frequently because it documented for the first time the ineffectiveness of outpatient treatment for obesity, and thereby led to a more realistic assessment of the problem and of the means for coping with it," Stunkard wrote in 1983. "These means are still limited."

Indeed, a few years before Stunkard made that statement, a study published in the *International Journal of Obesity* had concluded that the effectiveness of weight-loss interventions had changed very little in the twenty years since Stunkard and McLaren-Hume published their 1959 review, and that "weight losses produced by different methods, from behavior therapy to anorectic medication, are very much the same."[4]

Over the ensuing decades, research has continued to support those findings.[5] A 1992 NIH panel found that after completing weight-loss programs, 90 to 95 percent of people generally regain as much as two-thirds of the weight they lost within one year and almost all of it within five years.[6] Those conclusions were the result of a "technology assessment conference" that looked at the state of the science on intentional weight loss more than thirty years after Stunkard and McLaren-Hume's seminal paper.

The fact that the NIH panel reviewed the best available science to date in 1992 and came up with essentially the same findings as their 1959 counterparts suggests that despite decades of supposed advances in weight management, the human body remained stubbornly resistant to sustained, intentional weight loss. In fact, a number of experts on the NIH panel made the point that Americans were now fatter on average than they had been in the 1960s—this despite the huge percentage of people who were trying to lose or maintain weight, and despite the massive diet industry (which in 1992 was worth more than $30 billion, less than half what it is today).

By that time, some weight-loss researchers were getting fed up that success rates for intentional weight loss seemed not to have budged since Stunkard and McLaren-Hume's day, and they wanted to believe those numbers were not really accurate. Because nearly every study on the long-term outcomes of weight-loss interventions had been conducted in formal hospital or university settings, the argument went, the results might not apply to the general public; people who enroll in these kinds of structured programs may be the toughest cases, with the least likelihood of success. So in 1993, two researchers started tracking down people who had "succeeded" at weight loss without necessarily being part of any formal study or program.

It's fair to say that those researchers, Rena Wing and James O. Hill, were (and still are) heavily invested in diet culture. Wing has published more than 200 scientific articles on the treatment and prevention of "obesity," and one of her titles is director of the Weight Control and Diabetes Research Center at the Miriam Hospital in Providence, Rhode Island. Hill founded a weight-loss program, wrote a diet book, and served on the NIH panel that developed the U.S. guidelines on "obesity." Like anyone who's built their career on the foundation of diet culture, they had a vested interest in trying to prove that, contrary to decades' worth of scientific evidence, intentional weight loss works.

Wing and Hill called their project the National Weight Control Registry (NWCR). The criterion for enrollment was that registrants had to have lost a significant amount of weight and kept it off for more than a year. The NWCR received financial support from drug companies, among other sources.[7] (Remember the role that pharmaceutical companies played in creating the "obesity epidemic" around the same time in order to promote drugs such as fen-phen? After that damning 1992 NIH report, it makes sense that they would want to invest in giving people hope that intentional weight loss works.) Wing and Hill began enrolling people, and within five years they collected some 2,500 weight-loss "success stories." (Today they report this number is more than 10,000 people—but that's still less than 0.005 percent of all dieters.[8]) Wing told the *New York Times* that they started the registry "really to convince ourselves and convince the world that there are people who are successful, and then to learn from them....There is something very optimistic about this whole data set."

The reality, however, is far less hopeful. As dietitian Joanne Ikeda and colleagues wrote in a 2005 critique of the NWCR, 72 percent of enrollees were steadily regaining weight.[9] That's pretty normal at the one-year mark; although many people are able to maintain weight loss for a year or so, within three years the overwhelming majority have regained all the weight they lost—and often more.[10] And a large-scale 2015 study of more than 278,000 people found that within five years, the proportion of people who've regained all their lost weight (or more) is somewhere between 95 and 98 percent—right in line with Stunkard and McLaren-Hume's findings.[11] In fact, a 2007 meta-analysis of weight-loss studies found that people's weight usually reaches its lowest point somewhere around the six-month mark of any diet or "lifestyle change"; it then starts increasing at about one year, after which the rate of weight regain speeds up over time.[12]

On any diet or weight-loss program, "you can assume that the first six to twelve months are the weight-coming-off part, and then after that is the weight-coming-on-part," says Traci Mann, a psychology professor at the University of Minnesota whose 2015 book, *Secrets from the Eating Lab,* explores why diets almost always fail. "Anybody who says 'on this diet it's just going to come off and not come back' is lying. There's no such diet. That's just not the way it works."

Even the most optimistic research shows that "successful" participants will have maintained an average weight loss of just a few pounds after five years—and that's after gaining back *more than 75 percent* of the weight they initially lost.[13] Very few studies follow participants for as long as five years; in the ones that do, trajectories of weight regain suggest that people's weight will continue to increase once the follow-up period is over.[14] So when the NWCR made its criterion for "success" having lost weight and kept it off for at least a year, it was being quite generous with the definition. Call it optimism or call it bias from researchers under the sway of diet culture and the multibillion-dollar weight-loss industry—you decide.

As Mann explains, most diet studies are done in weight-loss clinics by researchers whose livelihood at least partly depends on those clinics. Thus "obesity" experts who study weight-loss programs have a lot to lose if their research shows those interventions don't work. They have a strong investment in maintaining the illusion that long-term intentional weight loss is possible, and that pursuing it is a worthwhile way to spend your time.

If any other product had such a sky-high failure rate, people wouldn't dream of wasting their time and money on it. There would be class-action lawsuits, and message boards filled with disgruntled customers complaining they'd been ripped off. Declining sales or government intervention would eventually get the product pulled from the market. People just wouldn't stand for it. But when it comes to weight-loss programs, we blame ourselves, again and again, rather than blaming the shoddy product that doesn't do what it's advertised to do. And that's how diet culture retains its power over us.

Diets Drive Weight Up over Time

Imagine a product that not only fails to deliver on its promises but does the *exact opposite* much of the time: a hairbrush that leaves your hair more tangled one out of every three times you use it; a bottle of water with a 50-50 chance of making you thirstier; a car that takes you *away* from your destination on two-thirds of your trips. This is what diets and "lifestyle changes" are; not only do they fail to produce sustainable weight loss, they tend to result in weight *gain* over time.

I want to be clear that I'm not saying weight gain is bad; as we'll discuss in Chapter 5, being at a higher weight hasn't been shown to cause health problems (although it may be *associated* with some negative health outcomes), and weight *stigma* is likely a bigger risk to your well-being than weight itself. Despite what diet culture has told us, there's nothing wrong with being at a higher weight. What I'm saying is that you deserve to know just how much diet culture is jerking you around and wasting your time—and it's a lot. The Life Thief is selling you a product that purports to do one thing but in fact is likely to do the reverse.

In a 2007 review, Mann and a team of researchers gathered up every previous study that had followed people on weight-loss programs for two to five years, and analyzed the results. Across all the studies, they found, one-third to two-thirds of dieters gained back significantly *more* weight than they'd lost.[15] A number of these studies showed that dieting consistently predicted future weight gain, regardless of a person's body size when they started out (and the researchers also controlled for other potential confounding variables such as physical activity, baseline eating habits, and education level). As Mann and her coauthors explained, the studies they reviewed are biased toward showing more successful outcomes for dieting; given their very low follow-up rates, the studies lack data from people who gained back large amounts of weight and then dropped out. Also, after the study periods ended and participants were allowed to go off the particular diets being studied, many of these people went on *other* diets and experienced some short-term weight loss, likely reducing the amount of weight regain documented in the studies. In light of all this bias, the effectiveness of diets is undoubtedly even *worse* than the dismal results shown in the data. The only thing diets are really good at is causing people to gain weight over time.

"That's likely why I'm the size I am now—a couple decades of dieting," says Substantia Jones, a photographer and fat-acceptance activist who now identifies as "a happily fat woman" but spent her youth trying to shrink her body. "Each time I would of course lose weight and then gain it back with a divi-dend, so I ended up bigger and bigger each time," she says. When she finally stopped dieting and regained weight for the last time, her weight stabilized—and has not fluctuated signifi-cantly since.

I've heard from hundreds of people who've gone through this experience: intentionally lose weight, then gain it back plus some, ending up heavier than they started. When they realize the staggering failure rate of diets, most people are upset about how much time they wasted on an intervention that failed to do what it was supposed to. That reaction is understandable; it's infuriating that diet culture sells us this faulty product and then blames us when it doesn't work, often causing the precise thing—weight gain—it was supposed to "fix." "It's a brilliant business model, isn't it?" Jones says. "It keeps people coming back to the diet industry over and over again, and never at any point do we stop and think that it's their fault."

When people first learn that diets drive up weight over time, they sometimes get angry at *themselves* for having been duped by diet culture; might their lives be better, they wonder, had they never gained additional weight from dieting? Not necessarily, as Lisa DuBreuil can attest. Now a psychotherapist who treats eating disorders and addiction, DuBreuil was born the same year Twiggy became a fashion icon (1966) and grew up in a culture dominated by a thinner-than-ever beauty ideal. DuBreuil pursued that ideal throughout her youth in a series of diets that inevitably led to rebound bingeing and weight gain, but she doesn't see the latter as a bad thing. "Even though I'm in a much larger body now—you know, very fat—I like my body so much better and I'm so much more connected to and appreciative of my body than I was when I was growing up," she says. "Weight loss doesn't heal people from their internalized weight stigma. Bad body image is not cured by weight loss."

The research is clear in that regard. A 2018 study, for example, found that people's internalized weight stigma didn't budge even when they lost significant amounts of weight.[16] For DuBreuil, as for most people, learning to love and care for her body had nothing to do with shrinking it. As we'll discuss in Chapter 10, there are plenty of things you can do to take care of your body at *any* size—and they're all dramatically more effective than dieting.

Why Don't Diets Work?

We now know that diets don't work, but why? Chalk it up to our genes and brains. Research indicates that our bodies have a weight "set point" that they're genetically programmed to maintain—although it's really better described as a weight set *range* that spans a few sizes our bodies can be throughout our adult lives, depending on our circumstances.[17] (That is to say, your weight isn't meant to stay at the exact same number on the scale, despite what diet culture may have led you to believe.) Although our genes determine this set range, it can be changed through dieting—but not in the way you might think. When you repeatedly try to force your body below its set range, it may eventually *increase* that range in order to protect you against future famines (aka diets). That's why up to two-thirds of weight-loss attempts result in long-term weight *gain*. Your body will then defend that new, higher set range just as valiantly as it did your original set range. (Again, I just want to pause and say that none of this is "bad"—or your fault. Diet culture may be screaming in your ear right now that this rebound weight gain is a terrible thing, but it's actually just your body *doing its job to keep you alive* in a situation of food scarcity. More on that in a sec.)

Our bodies' weight set ranges are as genetic as our heights: some 70 percent of individual differences in body weight are dictated by genes.[18] The weight set range is like the setting on a thermostat, and the thermostat itself is located in a brain region called the hypothalamus.[19] Our bodies are like heating and cooling systems that increase or decrease their energy output in order to maintain the setting. So strong is the power of this set range that if your weight drops below it, your brain senses danger and kicks off a series of biological changes to help you regain weight and prevent weight loss from occurring again. Those changes include reductions in the amount of the "fullness hormones" leptin, peptide YY, and cholecystokinin; increases in the amount of the "hunger hormone" ghrelin; lower overall energy output; and reduced activity in the thyroid and sympathetic nervous system, both of which help regulate metabolism.[20] When you're restricting your energy intake, your brain also increases the reward value of food and pushes you to eat more energy-dense foods—whereas that reward value goes down in situations of food abundance.

These changes are the biological drivers of a phenomenon I call the Restriction Pendulum, which is most people's natural reaction to deprivation. When the pendulum swings to the restriction side—which diet culture frames as "success" and "being good"—inevitably there's going to be a swing back in the other direction, because your body perceives restriction as dangerous. To your body, diets (or "lifestyle changes," or "eating plans," or whatever they call themselves now) feel like famine. Even the most seemingly gentle diet pulls the pendulum to the side of restriction. When that happens, your body's natural response is to push the pendulum back to the other side—to eating a *lot*, feeling out of control with food, even bingeing. A pendulum can't stop in the middle when it's been pulled to one side; it must swing in the opposite direction with equal force. Your body is exactly the same. It won't find stillness and peace until it has responded to the restriction.

Here's what that looks like in our lives: first we restrict, restrict, restrict (or "eat clean, eat clean, eat clean")...then we end up eating to the point of discomfort, often on foods that were deemed forbidden. And that makes us think we have no self-discipline, we're out of control, we simply can't be trusted to eat certain foods, we're uniquely broken while everyone else can have a bowl of ice cream without polishing off the whole carton. We berate ourselves as though what happened was about our minds, our lack of willpower. But it's not. It's physiological—a survival impulse encoded into your body.

When you get cold, you shiver. That's how your body keeps you warm so that you can survive. And when you're restricted or deprived of food, your body turns up the food-seeking signals *because it wants you to survive.* It pumps out the hunger hormones, turns down the fullness hormones, and lowers your metabolic rate, all in the service of keeping you from starving. This isn't a failure of your mind to control your body; this is your body taking care of you.

If you're bingeing in response to a diet, here's what I want you to know: Your body is not broken. *You are not broken.* You haven't irreparably damaged your hunger-and-fullness sensors. Your body is just trying to protect you. This is a natural, predictable, automatic response to famine—*and that's what diets are*. It's not you. It's not a defect. The Restriction Pendulum has allowed our species to survive, so we wouldn't be here without it. But we also don't need to spend our lives swinging on that pendulum anymore. To reclaim our time from the clutches of diet culture and reach our full potential, we need to get off the Restriction Pendulum. We need to stop pushing our bodies into starvation mode.

Throughout this book, I've talked about why *intentional* weight loss is neither effective nor sustainable. But what about *unintentional* weight loss? It really depends on the cause. If you inadvertently lose weight because something horrible happens in your life—illness, say, or the loss of a loved one—and you temporarily lose your appetite, the pendulum will most likely swing back once you recover, returning your weight to its genetically determined range. And let's all be grateful for that, because again, *we wouldn't be here on this planet right now* if human bodies were unable to bounce back from illness and psychological distress. In other cases, as when you heal your relationship with food, you may have some longer-term, unintentional changes in weight—but we don't know exactly what those changes will be. Some people's weight set ranges fall on the high end of the spectrum—the "overweight" and "obese" categories on the BMI chart—and there's absolutely nothing wrong with that: size diversity is a real thing, and people's body sizes are as heterogeneous as our height, hair and skin color, shoe size, and pretty much any other human characteristic you can think of.

For some people, though, making peace with food and learning intuitive eating and joyful movement (which we'll discuss in Part II) may result in some unintended weight loss. That certainly doesn't happen for everyone—many people experience some initial weight gain when they give up diet-culture behaviors, while others experience no change at all—and anyone who tells you that intuitive eating will inevitably bring weight loss is just selling you another diet. You can't know at the outset what will happen for you once you make peace with food (beyond the fact that your weight range will eventually stabilize *somewhere*), so you just have to trust that your body will arrive at its happy place, wherever that is, and let it do its thing. As much as the diet-culture part of your brain may want to know exactly how your size will change when you give up dieting, the truth is that no one can predict that. When it comes to finding a stable weight, our bodies are a hell of a lot smarter than our conscious minds.

Life as a Weight-Loss Unicorn

What about that tiny percentage of people who do maintain intentional weight loss, you might ask. Restriction (or "lifestyle changes" and diets by any other name) must be working for them, right? Not so much. Sure, they lose weight, but it's generally at the expense of the rest of their lives. That's evident in the research on members of the NWCR, who use behaviors to maintain weight loss that include weighing themselves compulsively, weighing and measuring food, not taking any breaks from their exercise routine, adhering to strict diets even on holidays and vacations, and basically having all of their time monopolized by their efforts at weight control. Even weight-loss advocates acknowledge what a sacrifice the people in the NWCR are making in service of weight loss. Kelly Brownell, founder of the Rudd Center for Food Policy and Obesity, said of the NWCR participants in 2011, "You find these people are incredibly vigilant about maintaining their weight. Years later they are paying attention to every calorie, spending [a long time every day] on exercise. *They never don't think about their weight.*"[21] (Emphasis added.)

When I was treating severe eating disorders in my private practice, I often saw people like this—people who never *didn't* think about their weight. Who organized their time around their eating and workout routines, often at the expense of family, friends, and hobbies. Who never deviated from that regimen, even on vacation. Who obsessively tracked calories, "macros" (or macronutrients), and the number on the scale. Whose entire lives were devoted to shrinking their bodies or maintaining their weight.

In eating-disorder-treatment circles, we have a word for these behaviors: *disordered.* When our clients are engaging in them, we work to help them stop. We encourage them to delete their calorie-tracking apps and get rid of their scales. We urge them to go out to restaurants with friends instead of eating weighed-and-measured meals at home alone. We help them replace their time spent on obsessive food and exercise routines with hobbies, friendships, and *life.*

Just because someone might start out in a larger body instead of a smaller one doesn't change the fact that organizing your life around weight-loss behaviors creates disorder in your relationship with food and everything else, diverting your time and mental energy from the things that really matter. No matter your size, if your life revolves around food, exercise, and your weight, there's a problem and you deserve help. Indeed, as a 2017 paper in the *International Journal of Eating Disorders* pointed out, "There are remarkable parallels between the behavioral patterns of successful weight loss maintainers from the NWCR and individuals with chronic anorexia nervosa."[22] Yet in diet culture, people in larger bodies who engage in these kinds of behaviors are applauded and held up as "success stories," even as their lives are being dominated by the pursuit of thinness.

That was very much the case for Glenys Oyston, who became a member of the NWCR in 2003. Oyston was one of those unicorns who had lost a significant amount of weight and kept it off for more than five years—sixteen years, in her case. Oyston started out with what she calls "light dieting" and was able to lose a fair amount of weight and keep it off, shrinking herself into the "normal" BMI category. But it got harder and harder to maintain that weight loss over the years, so she ramped up her dieting and exercise to an extreme degree. "This kind of restriction took me to a whole new level of food obsession that involved spending hours on the internet looking for ways to diet, searching for recipes, poring over nutrition data and facts, and looking at endless before-and-after photos of weight-loss 'successes,'" she says. "That's when I stumbled across the NWCR."

Oyston enrolled in the registry when her dieting was at its most restrictive and her weight was at its lowest point in her adult life. "I had kept the required amount of weight off for years by that point, so I figured why not be an example to the world?" she says. "I was so proud that I got to be in a registry for all my troubles and hunger." But that level of weight-loss obsession took over her life.

Oyston was in an unsatisfying relationship at the time. Rather than dealing with those issues head-on, however, she tried to fix them by shrinking her body—believing, as we're all taught to do in diet culture, that thinness would automatically lead to love and fulfillment. "I wasted years in a relationship that wasn't right for me *and* years feeling unhappy that my thin body wasn't making me feel as amazing as it was supposed to," she says. Meanwhile, her partner was frustrated because Oyston was so fixated on weight and food that it was hindering her ability to be present. "I really thought I was fixing the 'problem' of our relationship, but I was probably making it way worse," she says.

Compounding matters, she chose a professional path that allowed her to obsess about food and weight all day long and promised to keep her thin: she became a dietitian. Though today she's happy with that career choice (she has stopped dieting and has built a rewarding practice in the anti-diet niche), Oyston wonders if she might have pursued her childhood dream of becoming a writer if she hadn't been so caught up in maintaining her weight loss. "As for hobbies, I didn't have time for any of those," she says. "My hobby was dieting." For Oyston, as for so many people in that tiny percentage of dieters who can maintain intentional weight loss long-term, the pursuit of a smaller body eclipsed so many more important aspects of life. Weight loss was a full-time job.

The "Wellness" Trap

The Wellness Diet—the modern-day guise of diet culture—might seem like a more productive way to spend your time than on weight-loss attempts, because at least you're taking care of your health, right? But as we discussed previously, it's just as much of a waste of your time, energy, and other precious resources. Of course, prioritizing your health might be a value that you hold, and there's nothing wrong with that (although if it's *not* a value for you at this point, there's no shame in that, either—health isn't a moral obligation, nor is it within reach for millions of people for a lot of deep, systemic reasons that largely boil down to social injustice[23]). If you want to pursue health and you have the means to do it, great. But the Wellness Diet is full of dubious claims, unscientific assumptions, and wild conjectures that don't hold up under scrutiny, which means that chasing after this version of health is robbing you of time you could be spending on health-promoting behaviors that *actually work* (or, you know, the millions of other things you want to spend time on in life).

Take, for example, the supposed food-intolerance testing offered by many alternative- and integrative-health practitioners. One of the most common forms of this testing is a blood test to measure IgG (or immunoglobulin G) antibodies to specific types of food. These tests purport to diagnose "food sensitivities" that allegedly manifest as numerous disparate conditions such as acne, eczema, dry skin, bloating and other digestive issues, fatigue, joint pain, migraines, respiratory problems, weight gain (or difficulty losing weight), ear infections, and sinus infections.[24] The reactions to supposed IgG food sensitivities are usually described as being delayed or chronic, so it's not immediately obvious which food is "causing" the problems.

I'm using quotation marks and "supposed" here because IgG antibodies in the blood don't mean you have a food intolerance — in fact, quite the opposite. Pretty much anyone in good health has IgG antibodies to many different foods, and these antibodies have specifically been linked to the development of food *tolerance* or desensitization.[25] If your blood contains IgG antibodies to a wide variety of foods, it means you've been exposed to those foods and your body is totally cool with them. Yet too many "holistic" health practitioners continue to administer IgG tests and give people long, color-coded printouts of foods they're purportedly intolerant to, with no regard for the scientific evidence against this practice. They freak people out and cause them to restrict their eating unnecessarily, all under the guise of "wellness." The same is true for numerous other forms of testing embraced by the alternative-medicine field, among them hair testing, cell testing, muscle testing (aka applied kinesiology), skin-injection testing (aka provocation-neutralization testing), and electrodermal testing.[26] These tests, and the diets that practitioners prescribe based on their pseudoscientific results, are bogus — and a waste of time. (Meanwhile, elimination diets are often considered the "gold standard" for diagnosing food sensitivities, but they're problematic, too — more on that shortly.)

Another way in which the Wellness Diet wastes people's time is the current vogue for "anti-inflammatory" diets. Inflammation has become the latest bogeyman in chronic disease because it's been associated with health conditions such as heart disease, type 2 diabetes, and certain types of cancer. Inflammation is certainly a part of the disease process for many chronic diseases, but inflammation itself isn't necessarily the main culprit; often some underlying condition is both causing the inflammation and contributing to the development of disease. Because of the correlation, though, many medical professionals have begun to treat inflammation as though it *causes* disease; in some circles, reducing inflammation via supposedly anti-inflammatory foods has started to be seen as a panacea for treating and preventing disease. Unfortunately, there are multiple problems with that reasoning.

For one thing, the cardinal rule in statistics is that *correlation does not imply causation;* we can't infer that one thing causes another just because the two things are correlated. One of the classic examples of this is that male-pattern baldness is highly correlated with heart disease. So while it's probably very tempting for the hair-loss-treatment industry to advertise that its products prevent heart disease, in reality baldness does not cause heart disease at all; instead, a third factor—high testosterone—causes an increased risk of *both* baldness and heart disease. That means baldness is just a symptom, not a cause. Correlation does not imply causation.

In the same way, inflammation has been found to be *associated* with a number of different health conditions, but it hasn't been shown to *cause* them per se. Here are a few things that may be underlying causes of inflammation, according to a large body of research (see if you can spot the commonalities): lower social class, being divorced or separated from a partner, not having a job, being in financial trouble, having a greater number of negative interactions with other people, having people close to you struggle with their health, and being treated with disrespect or verbally threatened because of your race or your weight.[27] In other words, having bad shit happen to you—especially experiences of social injustice—is a risk factor for both increased inflammation and chronic disease. Another risk factor for chronic inflammation is weight cycling—repeatedly losing and regaining weight, which is what almost inevitably happens when people embark on weight-loss efforts. And when the true cause of inflammation is psychological distress, injustice, and yo-yo dieting, is eating more kale really going to help?

In fact, targeting inflammation through specific food choices or exclusions hasn't been conclusively shown to prevent or slow the development of disease or chronic inflammation.[28] We just don't have enough good scientific evidence to be able to claim with certainty that a particular way of eating is the ticket to a disease-free life via lower levels of inflammation, because there are so many confounding variables. All of the supposed anti-inflammatory diets that exist to date are based on speculation, because no food has definitively been shown to prevent disease by lowering inflammation in the human body over the long term, even if certain components in the food theoretically could.

What's more, the idea that people are personally responsible for reducing inflammation in their bodies by eating a certain diet conveniently passes the buck, distracting us from the real problem, which is sociocultural. If we really want to reduce people's levels of chronic inflammation in any significant way, we need public-health interventions that help end racism, weight stigma, and economic inequality. We need mental-health services that are accessible and affordable. We need to reduce the toll of chronic stress in people's lives, not give them one more thing to stress out about (namely inflammation) and one more supposed solution that's economically out of reach for most people (because green juices cost a lot of green).

Sure, regularly eating fruits and vegetables is associated with overall good health, and it's important to make these foods accessible to people of all socioeconomic backgrounds (another form of social justice) without linking that access to arguments about the so-called "obesity epidemic" (another form of weight stigma). But fruits and vegetables are not a panacea for preventing inflammation or disease—no food is.

Neither is any form of cleanse or detox, which is not only unnecessary and a waste of time but also potentially dangerous for both your physical and mental health. Cleanses and detoxes are based on a flawed understanding of human physiology claiming that your organs and digestive system need a "break" after eating particular foods. In reality, you don't need to deliberately do anything to "rest" or "reset" your organs: your digestive system, liver, and kidneys are self-cleaning. They're not like filters in the sink that get clogged with gunk and need to be cleaned out; they're more like a wastewater-treatment plant that uses chemicals to neutralize and dispose of harmful compounds. (Speaking of chemicals, they get a bad rap under the Wellness Diet, but your body is 100 percent chemicals—primarily oxygen, carbon, hydrogen, nitrogen, calcium, and phosphorus—and you'd die without them.) Like most things in your body, your liver, kidneys, and digestive system function just fine with no outside intervention. Unless you have a rare disease, these organs work for you 24/7 without your conscious control. You don't need to give your digestive system a "break" any more than you need to give your heart a break from beating or your lungs a break from breathing. Your body's *got this*.

What about when your body *hasn't* got this, as in cases of chronic disease? That's where the Wellness Diet and its false promises can be almost irresistible—and can lead to some extremely wild goose chases. Take the case of Katherine Zavodni, a fellow dietitian who treats eating disorders. Zavodni has ulcerative colitis, an autoimmune, inflammatory disorder of the large intestine that's notoriously hard to treat and can cause terrible pain and chronic diarrhea, as it did for her for many years. Standard medical treatments weren't working, and Zavodni was miserable—unable to leave the house, pooping more than a dozen times a day, and in constant pain. At this low point she went on an intense, months-long elimination diet under the guidance of an osteopath. She also tried acupuncture, weird powdered supplements that cost $60 a jug, and even quacky practices such as applied kinesiology. She spent years tumbling down the alternative-medicine rabbit hole—all to no avail. "None of it ever really seemed to make a damn bit of difference," Zavodni says. "It was just so demoralizing. I had worked so hard. And the default assumption when you experience something like that isn't 'This didn't work for me,' it's 'I must have done it wrong.'"

Of course there are people with legitimate food allergies and intolerances, such as peanut allergies or celiac disease, for whom avoiding certain foods really is a matter of self-care. But as we'll discuss shortly, most of the "autoimmune diets" and "chronic-disease diets" floating around today are just as much a part of diet culture as every other "plan," "protocol," or "program" out there. The past several years have seen a wave of books and blogs filled with sensational stories of people who've healed from debilitating diseases as a result of cutting out certain foods. Some of these stories are undoubtedly true—maybe even for you or someone you know. Yet for countless other people like Zavodni, eliminating foods never did anything but cause mental anguish; sometimes it even increased physical symptoms. Not only that, but disordered eating is a major cause of digestive distress in and of itself—and that often gets overlooked in diet culture's rush to point the finger at food.

Like so many people who have similar experiences with the Wellness Diet, Zavodni blamed herself instead of blaming the spurious methods used by the providers she'd seen, or blaming the providers themselves. "That's one of those incredibly perfect parallels with diet culture," she observes today. "It's like when the weight doesn't come off, [people say] 'I worked so hard—what did I do wrong?' That's where it leaves people. Blaming themselves." Promoters of the Wellness Diet, meanwhile, are likely to fan the flames of this self-blame. Zavodni describes the attitude of the alternative-health practitioners she saw: "If it doesn't work for you then you're too lazy, or you don't want to do this, or you don't have the willpower to make the changes, and that's on you. I have the solution—whatever is wrong with you, I can fix it—but you have to be willing to make a lifestyle change."

As an eating-disorder clinician, Zavodni knows how false and harmful the Wellness Diet's messages are to people's well-being. Yet sometimes, when her disease flares up and the pain is bad enough, she feels tempted to go down that road again— even today, years out from her fruitless journey into the world of elimination diets and bogus alternative treatments. (Zavodni's condition eventually did improve, thanks in part to numerous surgeries that removed affected parts of her colon.) "So much of the narrative that you hear now is 'I did the Whole30 and I felt so amazing,' and for somebody who has spent so much of my adult life feeling the very opposite of amazing, those narratives are still seductive to me," Zavodni says. "Not that I'm launching myself into the Whole30 diet—I've never done it, and I won't ever do it—but it seduces me sometimes, on my worst days. Like maybe there is some magical thing out there that I could be doing that would make all the difference in how I feel, because that's so much of what people are saying. I am acutely, painfully aware of how those messages harm us as a community and harm us as individuals, and still I sometimes wonder, *What if I eliminated gluten?* Or, *What if I eliminated all the things under the sun?*" The fact that Zavodni could be lured in like that, with all the knowledge and experience she has, both personally and professionally, "just shows how seductive and powerful those messages are."

The gluten issue is particularly insidious. The idea that people could have a low-grade intolerance or sensitivity to gluten has become a popular line of thinking thanks to the gluten-free trend. In reality, though, gluten intolerance (officially "non-celiac gluten sensitivity," or NCGS, in scientific literature) is often misdiagnosed or improperly self-diagnosed.[29] No biological marker identifies the condition, which means it cannot be diagnosed with a blood test or a stool sample: there's no way to tell from the outside whether or not someone has it, so any diagnosis of NCGS is based solely on people's self-reported symptoms in response to gluten, combined with tests to rule out celiac disease and wheat allergy. What's more, in many cases people's symptoms don't resolve on a gluten-free diet, and any genuine reaction to gluten-containing products may not be related to gluten at all.

To date, only a few randomized, controlled trials (RCTs, the most reliable form of study) have tested whether gluten is really the cause of people's symptoms. The best-designed of these studies, published in 2013, showed that when it comes to gluten, there's a strong "nocebo effect"—a phenomenon where merely *thinking* that something (such as gluten) is making you sick causes actual symptoms. (It's the opposite of a placebo effect, where believing that the placebo is making you better reduces your symptoms.) In the 2013 study, people weren't told whether they were getting gluten or not. But many of them thought they were getting gluten and *expected* to feel bad when eating it, so they did—even those who had in fact been given gluten-free food.[30] It didn't matter what they were actually eating. "It was just such a strong expectation that they were going to be receiving gluten at some point during their trial," says Jessica Biesiekierski, the lead author of the study. "I think they had built up such a sense of anxiety and expectation toward when they would feel those symptoms that they [attributed] to gluten."

Part of the difficulty with research like this, says Biesiekierski, is that there's no way to find people to study in NCGS trials who lack strong beliefs about gluten. The only way that researchers can get people into these studies is by finding folks who self-identify as having the condition—a confounding factor, because if you've already self-diagnosed with NCGS, you're more likely to be vulnerable to the nocebo effect with gluten. I asked Bie-siekierski whether, in light of her research, she thinks non-celiac gluten sensitivity is a viable diagnosis, or whether it even really exists. "I don't think that it exists," she says. "And if it does, it's likely to affect only a very, very small number of people." That's not to say that the people who believe they have NCGS don't legitimately have symptoms; they absolutely do. It's just that glu-ten doesn't seem to be the cause of those symptoms, whereas their *beliefs* about gluten do seem to play a role. "If somebody so strongly believes that something is going to be responsible for triggering their symptoms, then just that thought is enough sometimes," Biesiekierski says.

Regrettably, most people—including some health profes-sionals—don't know about the nocebo effect or Biesiekierski's findings on NCGS, so they continue to believe that gluten-free diets work for conditions other than celiac disease or wheat allergy. In recent years I've seen a dramatic increase in the num-ber of health professionals recommending a gluten-free diet for the management of autoimmune diseases such as Hashimoto's thyroiditis (which I happen to have) and lupus; in reality, how-ever, there's no convincing evidence to date that it's beneficial to go gluten-free for autoimmune diseases unless you *also* have celiac disease—which makes sense, because people with celiac disease should be avoiding gluten anyway. Nearly every study showing any benefit from a gluten-free diet for autoimmune dis-ease was conducted in people who *had celiac disease.* The results are therefore not generalizable to the non-celiac population.[31]

One study from 2014 did find that self-reported adherence to a gluten-free diet in people who had inflammatory bowel dis-ease (a type of autoimmune disease) was associated with greater self-reported symptom reduction even in those who *didn't* have celiac disease.[32] This wasn't an RCT, however, meaning we can't say that going gluten-free *caused* the symptom reduction. It's very likely that the self-reported benefits came from a nocebo effect, since these were people who, you know, live in the world and have heard the hype about gluten-free diets.

Ironically, the one piece of Biesiekierski's research that seems to have taken hold of the public imagination is that some people with so-called NCGS may instead be reacting to a different component of wheat and many other foods called FOD-MAPs. (The acronym stands for fermentable oligosaccharides, disaccharides, monosaccharides, and polyols—a group of short-chain carbohydrates that can cause a greater-than-average amount of gas when broken down in the intestines.) Some research indicates that doing a short-term low-FODMAP diet, followed by systematically increasing FODMAPs to identify any intolerances, may benefit some people with irritable bowel syndrome (IBS).* That's why Biesiekierski's team decided to put all of the participants in their 2013 study on a temporary low-FODMAP diet in order to isolate the effects of gluten and avoid any potential confounding from FODMAPs.

The past several years have seen an explosion of health professionals recommending low-FODMAP diets and people self-diagnosing with FODMAP intolerance and putting themselves on the diet (which was never meant for long-term use, but which unfortunately both laypeople and health professionals misinterpret as a long-term solution). Yet the concept of FODMAP intolerance has the same problems as NCGS: people are increasingly vulnerable to the nocebo effect with FODMAPs because of all the hype about them; many doctors prescribe FODMAP restriction haphazardly, without determining the real cause of patients' GI issues; the low-FODMAP diet hasn't been studied long-term; and the research we do have shows that it may have negative

---

* Before you get too excited about this diet, be aware that research indicates it has many potential complications. Further, the evidence in favor of low-FODMAP diets is not conclusive: both gut-directed hypnotherapy and yoga have been shown to be equally effective for IBS symptoms.[33]

consequences on people's overall intestinal health by reducing levels of beneficial bacteria.[34]

More troubling, for people who are vulnerable to disordered eating—which includes the vast majority of American women and an increasing number of people of other genders—cutting out gluten or FODMAPs can mask or exacerbate disordered-eating behaviors such as restriction, food fears, and unnecessary food avoidance. Those disordered behaviors, in turn, can further aggravate functional gut disorders (FGDs)—gastrointestinal problems such as IBS, heartburn, constipation, diarrhea, and bloating, which are not caused by structural issues with the gut. FGDs affect up to 98 percent of people with eating disorders,[35] which makes complete sense: disordered-eating behaviors of any kind wreak havoc on the digestive system. Research has also shown that disordered eating can cause increased sensitivity in the gut, which may in turn cause people to have a heightened perception of sensitivity to certain foods.[36] Not only that, but among the general population of patients seeking help for FGDs and other gastrointestinal issues, up to 44 percent exhibit disordered-eating behaviors.[37] This is both because disordered eating can cause or exacerbate underlying GI problems and because people with GI disorders often eat in restricted ways to treat their conditions, which can lead to the development of disordered eating in and of itself. Whatever the case may be, people who restrict food components such as FOD-MAPs are at heightened risk of eating disorders—and the more stringent they are with that restriction, the higher the risk. As a 2019 study put it, "Strict adherence [to] a low-FODMAP diet should raise the suspicion of a possible underlying eating disorder."[38]

Let me just pause here and say that if you truly feel Wellness Diet methods such as cutting out gluten, FODMAPs, or other foods have worked for you—with no negative effects on your health or your relationship with food—then I'm happy for you.

Truly. You might just be one of the lucky ones for whom this stuff turns out all right.

The problem, though, is that for all of us—including those "wellness" unicorns—who venture down the road a ways into the Wellness Diet, the concept of diet culture tends to take on a larger meaning. Your diet often *becomes* your culture, replacing other forms of culture in your life. Instead of spending time with friends and family, you're spending time on meal prep and complex dietary restrictions. Rather than going to see a play or a concert, you're watching Netflix documentaries about the foods that are supposedly going to kill or save you. In lieu of reading about politics or the arts or social causes—or just curling up with a good novel—you're reading about food, nutrition, and health.

I know that feeling all too well. As a young journalist, I was so fixated on those topics that I made them my main focus, my full-time beats. I created a career for myself that allowed my obsession to flourish—a career that gave me at least eight hours a day to spend researching and reading all about organic farming, gluten-free diets, fiber, protein, and even, occasionally, eating disorders. (Sadly, in reporting a short piece about orthorexia in 2006, it never dawned on me that the term perfectly described my relationship with food at the time.) The obsession didn't end with my workdays, though; often I would stay awake until 2 a.m. doing research that I told myself was for work but was really my desperate attempt to control my own health (and, of course, to lose weight—though by that point I didn't want to admit it, for fear of seeming uncool to my foodie friends). My early career choice was ultimately an attempt to get a handle on my food issues, to master this demon that had caused me so much pain. Yes, it was partly motivated by a covert desire to shrink my body. But it was also an effort to untangle my disordered behavior with food—and, in a larger sense, to find a sense of control in this unpredictable world.

For anyone who has lost years of their life to dieting and the disordered pursuit of wellness, we must have compassion—and that includes compassion for ourselves. We all want to be happy, accepted, and loved, which is what diet culture promises we'll achieve through thinness and "perfect" eating. We all want to avoid disease and live long, fulfilling lives. We all want to feel good in our bodies.

Diet culture holds out the promise of giving us these things, if only we achieve its version of "wellness"—which of course is thin, young, able-bodied, wealthy, and usually white and cisgender as well. Through media, advertising, health care, and conventional wisdom, diet culture constantly reinforces the notion that eating and moving your body in a Wellness Diet–approved way will lead to happiness, success, acceptance, and love. Unfortunately, in the effort to make our lives longer and healthier by diet culture's standards, we *lose* an untold amount of life to the pursuit of health and wellness. Our efforts to extend our time on this planet end up sucking it away. Once again, diet culture fails to keep its promise.

CHAPTER 4

How Diet Culture Steals Your Money

Linda Aubuchon, a communications and PR professional in Detroit, Michigan, estimates that she has lost at least $200,000 to diet culture. Now in her late forties, Aubuchon started her first formal diet in college, when her parents paid for her to go on NutriSystem. "Since then, it's just been a never-ending parade of every conceivable program, pill, and book out there to control my weight," she says.

Each formal weight-loss program she tried cost at least $1,000, not including the price of the special foods she had to buy for most of them. None of those programs produced long-term results. After giving birth to her son, Aubuchon became more extreme in her dieting behaviors to lose her pregnancy weight. Now she was not only following yet another diet but restricting her food intake to starvation levels and exercising compulsively every day. These disordered behaviors led to more weight loss than Aubuchon had ever experienced before, and it seemed like this time it was going to stick. "I felt very proud and accomplished, and I wanted to help people find the same success that I thought I had found," she says. So she decided to buy into a diet-program franchise — for the low, low price of $35,000. Of course, her motivation wasn't solely altruistic or entrepreneurial: "It was definitely in my mind that buying this franchise would be a way for me to further control and guarantee that I would never regain the weight," she says.

Spoiler alert: it wasn't the solution Aubuchon hoped for. At first she was relatively successful, both with her weight-loss maintenance and with the franchise. Soon, though, she started to realize that the diet program's business model was built on the fact that her clients would fail. "You make more money by having repeat customers," she says, explaining what the franchise's head office told her. "They didn't say you're going to do better if your customers fail, but they did clearly say that people will come back to you over and over again when they have the littlest bit to lose." That didn't sit well with Aubuchon, given her own history as a serial dieter. Meanwhile, she was experiencing one of the most common side effects of a restrictive diet and compulsive exercise: binge eating.

Seeking help with this issue, Aubuchon ended up in therapy with binge-eating expert Amy Pershing. (Aubuchon doesn't include the therapist's fees in her tally of the money she lost to the Life Thief, although treatment for disordered eating can definitely be one of diet culture's hidden costs.) The therapy focused not only on Aubuchon's eating issues and dieting history, but also on her life values and career goals. Through that process, she ultimately decided to close her weight-loss franchise — at a significant financial loss, and without another job lined up — so that she would no longer have to build her business on the backs of fellow dieters.

For several years after that, Aubuchon made a real effort to break free from diet culture. But she never completely let go of it; she wasn't ready. Life got in the way. She went through a divorce — partly because of the financial problems that her investment in diet culture had caused — and ended up gaining even more weight. This led to a decision to have weight-loss surgery, even though her insurance wouldn't cover it because her weight wasn't high enough to be deemed a case of "medical necessity." She paid out of pocket.

Aubuchon chose to get the laparoscopic band (aka "lap

band"), a type of weight-loss surgery that involves putting a silicone band around the stomach and filling it with an adjustable amount of saline fluid to squeeze the organ. The lap band is supposedly less invasive and more gentle than other forms of surgery such as gastric bypass, where part of the stomach is removed, but Aubuchon still had complications right from the start. "The band for me was never the tool that it was promised to be," she says. "I lost a little weight, but I really struggled with just living with the band." Loath to spend more money and endure more surgery to reverse the band, she ultimately had all the fluid removed — so the band is still there, but no longer constricting her stomach. She then made one final, last-ditch attempt at Weight Watchers (even though she'd tried it unsuccessfully before) and is now trying to recover for good from her disordered eating.

In the end, Linda Aubuchon spent a fortune without any long-term success at losing weight and keeping it off — and it certainly wasn't for lack of trying. Her experience might be more extreme than the average person's, but it's not atypical. Millions of Americans spend their hard-earned cash on weight-loss efforts every year, with little to show for it. As noted previously, in 2019 the research firm Marketdata reported that the U.S. diet industry is now worth more than $72 billion — a record high.[1] This number includes money spent on almost anything you can think of related to weight loss: commercial weight-loss programs; diet soft drinks, artificial sweeteners, and diet foods; retail and multilevel-marketing meal replacements and shakes; over-the-counter diet pills and prescription diet drugs; medically supervised diets and hospital-based weight-loss programs; bariatric surgery and related counseling; diet books and exercise videos; and gym and health-club revenues. (Remember that last one the next time you find yourself thinking that people join gyms for health rather than for weight loss.) And whereas sales of weight-loss products and foods are in decline, sales of weight-loss *services* are growing, poised to become the core of the market. Bariatric surgery is one of the most lucrative surgical specialties, with procedures costing $15,000 to $25,000 on average, according to the National Institute of Diabetes and Digestive and Kidney Diseases. Overall the weight-loss industry is expected to continue growing steadily, at a rate of 2.6 percent per year.

Adding Up the Hidden Costs

Think of all the ways you've participated in the diet-culture economy over the course of your life. Even if you've never been on a commercial diet plan like the $1,000 programs Aubuchon cycled through, how many "lite" and "guilt-free" foods have you bought over the years? How many weight-loss books, gym memberships, protein supplements, meal-replacement shakes? What about "shapewear" designed to make you look thinner, or cellulite creams and other snake-oil products that were supposed to somehow remove fat from your body? If you added up all the small sums you've spent trying to shrink yourself into society's unattainable ideal, you'd probably be looking at a minimum of a few thousand dollars, if not tens of thousands or more.

That includes a lot of costs you probably don't think of as tied to diet culture. For example, there's a protein bar that costs nearly $3 and contains as much fiber as several bowls of bran cereal; I won't name it because I don't want to give the brand additional business, but I'd never heard of this bar until I started treating eating disorders, and then suddenly I was seeing it daily in my clients' food logs. It's definitely diet food; claiming it was created to help end "obesity," the manufacturer urges you to reach for one of its bars in place of a muffin or a cookie. This type of bar is considered "safe" by people suffering with eating disorders, meaning that the critical, food-shaming voices in their heads don't berate them for eating this particular snack the way they would for eating something with, say, more calories or less fiber. (Foods that people with eating disorders consider safe are generally the exact same foods marketed for weight loss or "wellness" to the general population—just one of the many reasons why the line between dieting, subclinical disordered eating, and diagnosed eating disorders can be so blurry.) I've had clients who've spent a few thousand dollars a year on this one type of protein bar *alone*. Everyone needs to spend some money on food, of course, but diet foods are often much more expensive than other things you could be eating. Not to mention the fact that people often feel compelled to spend money on food that isn't truly satisfying because it's "acceptable" to diet culture. As many of my clients discover when they move into eating-disorder recovery, the diet foods they once thought of as delicious treats taste *terrible* compared with the many nondiet options they now allow themselves.

Speaking of eating disorders, the treatment for those is incredibly costly. Residential treatment programs cost around $30,000 per month, and many people with eating disorders stay for months at a time and go back more than once. These programs often don't accept insurance, and even for the ones that do, the co-payments can be sky-high. Meanwhile, outpatient treatment for eating disorders (which includes weekly or biweekly appointments with a therapist and a dietitian, plus regular monitoring by a medical doctor) can run $15,000 to $45,000 per year—again, much of it not covered by insurance. And some clients struggle with these disorders for years, racking up treatment bills in the hundreds of thousands and going deep into debt, since very few people have savings that can cover those kinds of bills.

That's of course if they're privileged enough even to get a diagnosis—the majority of people who struggle with disordered-eating behaviors are never diagnosed and never get treatment.[2]

One of the main reasons so few people get diagnosed is a pervasive stereotype born of diet culture: that people need to be emaciated in order to qualify as having an eating disorder. In reality, most eating-disorder sufferers are in the "normal" BMI category or above; by one estimate, as many as 30 percent of people seeking weight-loss treatment meet the clinical criteria for binge-eating disorder.[3] According to a 2015 report by the health care–focused investment firm Coker Capital Advisors, the eating disorder–treatment industry is a roughly $3.5 billion operation.[4]

These treatment costs aren't counted in the $72 billion that Americans spend on the diet industry every year, but most of that $3.5 billion should be added to the overall toll of the Life Thief. Why? Because the majority of people suffering with eating disorders (or significantly disordered eating that doesn't meet diagnostic criteria but still requires treatment) wouldn't be in this position without diet culture. Obviously not every eating disorder is caused by dieting; eating disorders have a multifaceted etiology that's part biological, part psychological, and part sociocultural (which is where diet culture comes into play). Still, dieting is generally recognized as a major risk factor; dieters' risk of developing an eating disorder can be eighteen times higher than nondieters'.[5]

Almost every client I've seen for disordered eating says their food issues began with an effort to lose weight or "eat healthier." Many were also previously shamed for their weight or praised for losing weight—both common triggers for eating disorders. "To end eating disorders we have to end weight stigma and thin privilege," says Amy Pershing, the psychotherapist and binge eating–disorder expert whom Aubuchon saw early in her recovery. Or, as sociologists Sharlene Hesse-Biber and colleagues put it, "Eating disorders are the logical conclusion of extreme self-imposed body control to attain a cultural ideal of ultra-thinness."[6] Go far enough down the road of dieting and it will end in a full-blown eating disorder. Diet culture's impossible standards for bodies—and the unearned privileges that come with being in a smaller body in this culture at this particular point in history—are a driving force behind the development of disordered-eating patterns. Until we eradicate diet culture, our chances of preventing eating disorders at the population level are pretty much nil.

The Price of "Wellness"

The Life Thief's financial toll further increases if we include all the sneaky manifestations of diet culture that have emerged since the turn of the millennium: "wellness" products and services such as cleanses and detoxes; "clean-eating" books; trendy "superfoods"; and elimination diets for the general population (rather than for people with a genuine food-allergy diagnosis or celiac disease). One wellness-industry research firm reports that the worldwide market for "healthy eating, nutrition, and weight loss" is worth a staggering $648 billion.[7] The North American cold-pressed juice market alone is expected to reach $311 million by the end of 2024.[8]

Katie Dalebout, creator of the book and podcast *Let It Out* and a survivor of orthorexia, knows a thing or two about how the Wellness Diet gobbles up money. When she discovered the wellness world during college, it quickly became her only hobby—and the organizing principle of her life. "I didn't really have any money, but all of my spending money went to going to the health-food store, or buying expensive superfoods and diet-disguised-as-wellness type foods on the internet," she says. Within a year, her orthorexic behaviors were so all-consuming (and her health so impaired) that she was diagnosed with an eating disorder. It stole her life for several years, damaging her health and depleting her bank account.

Dalebout would order expensive raw-vegan crackers, kale

chips, and other prepared foods from a trendy New York City restaurant she'd learned about on Instagram, then have them shipped to her apartment in Michigan. She once spent $20 on a "superfoods and herbs tonic"—basically a single-serving beverage. She bought raw, sprouted almond butter that cost at least that much per jar. Other people spent money on diet culture on her behalf, too: on weekend visits home, Dalebout got her mom to take her shopping at the health-food store so she could meal-prep for the week, and she persuaded her boyfriend at the time to buy all kinds of esoteric ingredients she'd learned about on wellness blogs, such as dulse, nutritional yeast, spirulina, and hemp seeds. "My graduation gift from college was a Vitamix," she says, referring to the fancy appliance prized by Wellness Diet acolytes for making smoothies and green juices. "That's what all my aunts and uncles pooled their money together for—to get me a $700 blender," she says.

Of Headlines and Panty Lines

Another stealthy way that diet culture can steal your money, beyond "official" diets and weight-loss plans, is mainstream health-and-fitness media that tout weight loss and foment fear about supposedly "bad" foods. If you've ever grabbed a magazine because of a cover line promising to help you "lose X pounds in X days"—if you've ever clicked on a headline like "The 10 Foods You Should Always Avoid"—you've put money in diet culture's coffers. This kind of messaging gets us to buy periodicals or give page views precisely because diet culture has led us to believe that thinness is the be-all and end-all of a healthy, happy life, and that we should be afraid of food because of its supposed power to diminish that life (whether by causing weight gain or by triggering more nebulous symptoms such as bloating, fatigue, or "brain fog"). And so it's a vicious cycle, where media outlets both respond to consumer demand for diet-related stories and perpetuate that demand by publishing them.

This insidious diet-culture rhetoric shows up in food media, too, with recipes for "guilt-free holiday desserts," "clean-eating" menus, and other moralizing ideas about food. Just as in women's magazines, these phrases pique readers' interest thanks to the saturation of diet culture. "I think we use the term *guilt-free* in media because it's effective," said Jacklyn Monk, managing editor at *WSJ.* (the *Wall Street Journal* magazine) and a longtime veteran of the magazine industry, in a panel discussion with me and two other journalists at the International Association of Culinary Professionals conference in 2018. Monk personally opposes this kind of messaging in media, but she acknowledges that it sells. "Unfortunately people click on it, and that means money, and then [editors are] told to repeat it." The tantalizing cover lines and clickbait headlines have also shifted over time, paralleling the shift in diet culture away from overt promises of weight loss and toward health-and-wellness rhetoric. " 'Lose X pounds in X days' was very common twenty years ago, and I think that is no longer the case," Monk said. "I think 'guilt-free' is maybe the new 'lose X pounds in X days.' "

The power of diet culture to sell products is likewise evident in the market for shapewear—undergarments and other clothes designed to make you look smaller and smoother. The shapewear industry is predicated on the idea that your body's natural curves and dimples are unsightly and need to be squished into submission, and it would seem that millions of people have bought into the hype. In 2012 *Forbes* magazine named Spanx creator Sara Blakely, then forty-one, the youngest self-made female billionaire.[9] Two years later, then–First Lady (and beloved female role model) Michelle Obama revealed that not only does she wear Spanx, but she "wear[s] them with pride."[10] Granted, in recent years the shapewear industry has faced some backlash from increasingly body-positive buyers who want comfort rather than constriction, and even from doctors who point out that the garments can pinch nerves and organs. Still, shapewear remains a huge market. Like diet culture in general, it has morphed and gone underground to keep pace with changing consumer tastes.

As the *New York Times* reported in 2015, Spanx and other shapewear companies responded to demand for greater comfort by developing new garments with less constriction and "just a subtle hint of shaping."[11] Not only that, but for a time the company included cards bearing feminist-inspired messages in every pack of "shaper shorts," and the back of the packaging read, "Re-shape the way you get dressed, so you can shape the world!" In reality, the thing being reshaped here is the discourse about why people should buy these products. Just as with other aspects of diet culture, the shapewear industry is trying to downplay its overtly body-negative past in order to hold on to market share—in this case, by co-opting feminist language.

Marketing and "Aspirational" Dieting

When diet culture steals our money, it's not simply a matter of individual choice—at least not entirely. We don't make those choices in a vacuum; they're conditioned by the culture we're born into, as well as by massive industries that cajole and coerce us into buying products that promise to "fix" the problem of our bodies. Kaila Prins, a content-marketing manager and host of the podcast *Your Body, Your Brand,* puts it this way: "You can't have diet culture without marketing." Marketers of everyday products psychologically profile us in order to influence us. These days they do it with such sophisticated means that we're often unaware of how their marketing is shaping our actions—yet it absolutely is. Linda Aubuchon never would have shelled out tens of thousands of dollars for commercial weight-loss programs if she hadn't been convinced that shrinking her body was the key to a happy life. No recent college grad would dream of asking her family for a $700 blender if it weren't for blogs and social-media messages lauding it as the must-have appliance for any healthy home. We'd never spend a *dime* on diet culture if we hadn't been conditioned to think it was a good investment—or at least worth the gamble for a potentially huge payoff. "There are these constant messages that you will benefit from doing this, and not just for your health," Prins says. Diet culture tells us that "you will get social capital, which is just as important as financial capital, and sometimes more important."

In fact, by leveraging the belief that a certain type of body will grant us social capital, diet culture is able to separate us from our financial capital. Tapping into consumers' internalized diet-culture beliefs is a great way for *any* company to squeeze money out of us—even businesses that have nothing to do with weight loss or "wellness." By associating their product with images of people who are thin, conventionally attractive, and outwardly fit and healthy (by diet culture's standards), companies can harness consumers' desires to *be* thin, conventionally attractive, fit, and healthy—with all the social currency and status those attributes confer.

Remember that diet culture is a system of beliefs that equates thinness with health and moral virtue, so the aspiration to be thin isn't just skin-deep. At its most fundamental level, it's about the desire to be seen as good, lovable, and *enough*. It's about the desire to be special, and the desire to belong. By using promises of weight loss and images of thin people to sell stuff, from diets to deodorant, companies are subtly transmitting the message that buying their product will give you all these deeper things that you truly want (and that all human beings deserve, no matter our appearance). Is it any wonder we buy in?

People can be seduced by the steady drip of diet-culture marketing even if they don't read fashion magazines or follow celebrities on Instagram. Take Lindley Ashline, for example: Now a body-positive photographer, Ashline grew up in a small, rural Southern town in the 1990s; she wasn't allowed to watch TV or read teen magazines, so she had very little exposure to pop culture or fashion. But she still absorbed plenty of toxic beliefs from diet culture, she says, notably the idea that "my body is terrible. It was just this underlying guilt about my body."

Ashline didn't think she could change her size or shape, so she never considered dieting. But then she hit puberty and went through the weight gain that people typically experience in that stage of life, and suddenly her body loathing reached a new level. She started to fantasize about dieting, about shrinking the body that felt increasingly unacceptable. But she grew up in a family that she describes as lower-middle-class or working-class, and as soon as she began to think about dieting she became acutely aware that it was out of reach for her financially. She and her family couldn't afford diet foods, meal replacements, or costly weight-loss-program memberships. "And so it became a life goal," she says. "It was very much this aspirational thing: *Someday when I have the money, I'm going to diet and then I'll be thin and acceptable.*"

Dieting as a class marker is a natural extension of diet culture: if you have money (but not the kind of body held up as the "ideal," which almost no one has anyway), you spend it on shrinking yourself, thereby earning your acceptability. Today the nuances are different than they were when Ashline was growing up, because it's no longer cool to be *dieting* per se. Now it's all about "wellness," and with that comes those expensive kale smoothies, grain-free crackers, and fitness classes — not to mention elimination diets such as the Whole30, which remove access to staple foods (bread, pasta, rice) that would otherwise provide nourishment and energy for a relatively low cost.

It's certainly possible to add more fruits and vegetables to your life without breaking the bank (and without driving yourself to the point of disorder). Yet "wellness" is a rarefied pursuit that's about much more than making small changes in your eating habits. Its logical conclusion is Gwyneth Paltrow selling $66 jade "yoni eggs" that supposedly give your vagina magical wellness vibes, alongside $50 jars of "biofermented" smoothie powder. Straight-up dieting, meanwhile, has lost its cultural cachet. "I think now dieting has become a class marker in the opposite direction," Ashline observes. "If you're dieting, you don't get it. You haven't caught on that that's not what we do nowadays— now it's lifestyle change." The same goes for brands; today, companies that sell frozen diet entrées or advocate calorie counting are seen as behind the times, unfashionable, and low-status.

This shift is part of a larger trend in consumerism. Cultural elites now signify their wealth by "inconspicuous consumption"— consumer-economy researcher Elizabeth Currid-Halkett's term for spending money on comparatively small luxuries such as organic free-range chicken, heirloom tomatoes from the farmers' market, and yoga and Pilates classes. Currid-Halkett explains that the modern "aspirational class" eschews overt manifestations of wealth—designer handbags or flashy cars—in favor of subtler purchases that convey knowledge and social status (many of which happen to be very much in line with the Wellness Diet). "In lockstep with the invoice for private preschool comes the knowledge that one should pack the lunchbox with quinoa crackers and organic fruit," she writes. "Knowing these seemingly inexpensive social norms is itself a rite of passage into today's aspirational class."[12] Following the Wellness Diet, then, is a type of virtue signaling that people use to secure and maintain their own class status.

Katie Dalebout remembers getting caught up in that ritual when she was struggling with orthorexia. "It became performative, like keeping up with the Joneses in a wellness way," she says. Dalebout followed other "wellness" people on Instagram and kept tabs on what they were eating or not eating, trying to emulate them and build her own following as a wellness influencer. When she saw someone blending more herbs into their "tonic" than she did, she felt compelled to add even more to her own, perpetuating a sort of herbal arms race that ended with her drinking a concoction that tasted terrible but cost thirty bucks. She then posted a picture of it, listing all the ingredients — thereby drawing her followers into the competition, too. When sharing pictures of food, she would include captions such as "post-yoga lunch" or "post-hike breakfast" to publicly declare she was "earning" her food through exercise. It didn't strike her as dieting, but that's exactly what it was — the Wellness Diet.

This competitive, performative element is certainly present in traditional dieting, too; we all know people who compulsively list their fitness accomplishments and scrutinize the bodies of everyone they meet to see how they compare. Most of the clients I treat for disordered eating tell me they eat less in public because they want to appear healthy and "good" in front of other people. If they don't come out ahead in these body comparisons or perform the "right" way of eating around others, they feel like they have "failed."

That's another trick of the Life Thief: the myth of personal failure, which says it's your fault if you don't do things by diet culture's standards. This myth conveniently also keeps people coming back and spending more and more money on interventions that don't work. Diet culture makes you feel like it's *your* fault — like if you were the kind of person you wanted to be, you'd be able to lose weight and keep it off. All those thin people you see in diet ads — jumping around with their kids in a park under a halo of sunshine, or hosting effortless dinner parties in their perfectly landscaped backyards — are able to do it, diet culture implies. So why can't you? Maybe you just aren't trying hard enough! After all, those people are just like you, so the only thing standing in your way must be *you*.

Or so the story goes.

So you keep buying the product (or different versions of the same thing) and hoping for a better result, thinking you simply need to work harder. But what if the product is destined to fail no matter what you do?

Opportunity Cost

In late 2009, soon after my colleagues and I were all laid off from our jobs at *Gourmet* when the magazine folded, I went to the unemployment office in Brooklyn to sign up for benefits while I figured out my next move. I'd read somewhere that in addition to covering a percentage of the salary from a lost job, unemployment benefits included tuition reimbursement in some cases. I was already enrolled in an expensive night program at NYU to get my master's in public-health nutrition and my registered dietitian's license; as luck would have it, I lost my job less than a month after the program started. So I figured I'd see if I could get some help paying for it.

When I told all of this to the unemployment officer, he basically laughed in my face. He explained there's no way they would cover it, because a career as a dietitian has a much lower earning potential than a career as a journalist (or at least it did at the time—a disparity attributable to the fact that dietetics is a female-dominated field). Unemployment benefits would cover education only in higher-paid fields than the one I was leaving. He sent me off with some printouts of earnings forecasts and a strong recommendation not to go down the dietetics path. I did so anyway—I was in too deep with diet culture to give up my dream of a career helping to end the "obesity epidemic," which I wholeheartedly believed in at the time—and ended up with a $250,000 student-loan debt that I'll be paying off for years to come.

Don't get me wrong—I'm not complaining about how things

turned out for me. I was ultimately able to bridge my two careers in a way I find fulfilling, and the combo has been able to financially support a middle-class life, student-loan repayments included. All things considered, I have a lot of economic privilege. Still, that experience in the unemployment office stuck with me. Years later, I wondered: *How many other people have traded in promising, satisfying careers for less-remunerative positions in the health-and-wellness field because diet culture has made them so obsessed with nutrition and fitness?*

Quite a few, it turns out. Having landed in the field of disordered eating, I now know dozens of colleagues who admit they went into careers in nutrition, personal training, or some other aspect of health and wellness because of their own issues with food; in so doing, they closed the door on career options that might have been more lucrative and fulfilling. (Not to mention less potentially harmful to their mental and physical health; working in the health-and-wellness field when you have your own issues is risky, both for yourself and for your clients.) For many of us, diet culture captured our imaginations at moments when our careers were malleable. We may have had bigger dreams, or other things we wanted to do, but we got waylaid by the Life Thief.

Kristie Amadio is one of those people. As a kid she started competing in weight lifting, and by age fourteen she had become an elite athlete, training for the Olympics in her home country of Australia. Weight lifting is a sport with weight classes, which meant that athletes were encouraged to keep a close watch on the scale; for Amadio, that spiraled into an eating disorder that persisted through her twenties and changed the trajectory of her life. When she retired from weight lifting at age twenty, she says, "my immediate thought was, *How can I maintain this body weight in this size and shape when I'm not doing elite-athlete exercise and training anymore?* It even had me choose the career that I went into once I left weight lifting." Amadio decided to become a wilderness instructor, in part because she loves the outdoors, but mostly because she wanted a way to keep her body from changing. "I thought to myself, *How can I get paid to exercise?* Essentially, *How can I have a functional eating disorder and get paid for it?*"

Not everyone whose career is shaped by their disordered relationship with food is quite so deliberate about the choice. In many cases it's a matter of getting pulled into the health-and-fitness world bit by bit. "If you go online right now and post a before-and-after picture of yourself, you will be inundated with people not just congratulating you but asking you how you did it," Prins, the content-marketing manager, says. "So suddenly you go from being the person who bought the program or bought the fitness classes to the person who is an expert—and then you see that there is capital to be gained. You say, 'People see me as an expert in my body, and they think I can be an expert in their bodies, so all I have to do is spend five thousand bucks on the nutrition certification or personal-trainer certification, and then I can make tens of thousands of dollars like these other coaches online.'" It's an enticing proposition.

That happened to Melissa Toler, a pharmacist who worked in the pharmaceutical industry and got involved in fitness competitions on the side. Eventually she became so passionate about weight loss and "wellness"—and had so many people seeking her advice on how to change *their* bodies—that she made it her career. Toler became certified as a health-and-wellness coach in 2013. When she was laid off from her pharmaceutical job a few months later, she didn't look for another one. "I left a very lucrative career, a six-figure-salary job," Toler says. "When my financial planner saw how much money I had made that year and that I was leaving [the industry], he said, 'You must really want to do this!'"

And she did. "You couldn't tell me anything different," she says. "I had a coach that I was paying a zillion dollars to help me do this. And thank God I had a lot of money saved up and I got a severance package and all that great stuff, so I had a cushion." She also was single without any dependents, so it seemed like a good time to make the leap.

Though Toler constantly saw people on the internet bragging about how they'd made six-figure incomes (or more) with online coaching businesses, the reality for her was very different. In part, she says, that's because "I didn't anticipate that my thinking would shift and I would be steered away from weight loss." As she healed from her own disordered relationship with food and her body, the cognitive dissonance of telling other people to shrink themselves got to be too much. She had to stop.

For Toler, trying to make a living as a wellness coach who wasn't selling diet culture's version of wellness had proven difficult. "The money was not what I thought it was going to be," Toler said. Eventually she returned to her original career, though she still teaches online courses on the side.

Of course, there are exceptions who make bank in the wellness world—and that comes with a different kind of opportunity cost. Being a wellness "influencer" means sponsorships, affiliate deals, speaking gigs, and other lucrative perks. Blogger Jordan Younger, for example—whose story of rebranding after orthorexia was told in Chapter 2, and who is known as The Balanced Blonde today—sold more than a million dollars' worth of a five-day vegan cleanse program under her previous brand, The Blonde Vegan.[13] When you're in that position, it can be very hard to leave, even if you're deep in the throes of an eating disorder.

"If you stop doing the thing that's hurting you, you stop making money," Prins says. "You have to figure out a different way to support yourself—and that is terrifying, especially if you're not in a place where that's financially viable for you." That means many influencers stay in a career that's perpetuating their disorder, because trying to recover would mean losing money as well as social capital. If you're lucky enough to make it big in the wellness field, the price you pay is often your own well-being. The trade-off is literally your money or your life.

In her book *The Body Is Not an Apology*, Sonya Renee Taylor distinguishes between "best-interest buying," which reflects a commitment to radical self-love, and "detriment buying," which is driven by the feeling that you're flawed or not good enough as you are. The difference between these two types of spending is in the motivation behind them. The same product could be an example of best-interest buying for one person and detriment buying for another, depending on the intentions and beliefs each person has about the purchase.

That's a helpful distinction to keep in mind when it comes to anything you buy, and it's especially germane to why people become health-and-wellness professionals. Depending on your motivation, embarking on a training program for a wellness-based career could be best-interest buying or detriment buying. For me, enrolling in the NYU program to become a dietitian was initially a detriment purchase: it was all about buying into diet culture and feeding my disordered thinking about food and bodies. Somewhere along the way, though, my mind-set and motivation changed; by the time I paid the registration fee for my final licensure exam it was definitely best-interest buying, because by that point I was building a career that was strengthening my recovery and helping others heal. I'm not working to "end the obesity epidemic" the way I thought I would when I started out; instead, I'm helping people recover from diet culture and internalized weight stigma.

Paying for the "War on Obesity"

One of the arguments used to justify the "war on obesity" is that people in larger bodies supposedly have higher health-care costs due to their body size, resulting in higher Medicare and

Medicaid spending and thus a bigger burden on taxpayers. In reality, though, the costs attributed to "obesity" are grossly inflated: excess spending on health care in the United States has nothing to do with body size.[14] The U.S. has higher health-care spending than any other developed nation—even when adjusting for relative wealth, and despite having a healthier population than most—primarily because we have higher salaries for physicians, profit-hungry health-care and insurance companies, and expensive new technologies.

Whenever you hear someone arguing that "obesity" contributes significantly to those costs, it's because they're calculating the "cost of obesity" in an unjust and stigmatizing way: *any* money that people in larger bodies spend on medical care is attributed to their size—even if they're going to the doctor for a condition that thin people also get, like, say, the flu. The condition might have no connection to body size, yet still it gets blamed on "obesity." What's more, estimates of the "cost of obesity" omit a wide array of confounding variables that could explain the association between body size and health outcomes, including a history of yo-yo dieting, the toll of weight stigma, and access to high-quality and nondiscriminatory medical care.[15] All of these factors are independently associated with adverse health outcomes, as we'll discuss in the next chapter, and could go a long way toward explaining any excess health-care costs in larger-bodied people. Moreover, people in higher BMI categories are often subjected to greater testing and treatment simply because their size is considered a risk factor, whether they need those interventions or not.

Meanwhile, our tax dollars are being used to fund the ill-advised "war on obesity." In the 2017 fiscal year alone, the CDC's Division of Nutrition, Physical Activity, and Obesity gave nearly $50 million in funding to state programs aimed at reducing "obesity" rates and preventing chronic diseases. Granted, not all of that money went to programs explicitly demonizing larger bodies; some of it may have gone to programs that simply helped, say, increase people's access to fruits and vegetables, with no weight-loss rhetoric attached. Still, nearly every nutrition and physical-activity program in diet culture comes with a side of weight stigma, so it's likely that the vast majority of these programs did, too.

I'm not against government spending on public-health initiatives—far from it. In general, evidence-based public-health programs have the potential to help address the extreme health disparities in this country and improve people's health and quality of life. I've worked on governmental public-health initiatives in the past and have friends who still do. What I take issue with is government spending on programs that spread diet-culture messages and stoke fears about the so-called "obesity epidemic": not only are such efforts ineffective, but they can cause a lot more harm than good to people's well-being. Like the war on drugs, the "war on obesity" further stigmatizes people who are already marginalized in our society, and does very little to promote health and well-being.

Indeed, as you're about to see, diet culture is terrible for your health.

CHAPTER 5

How Diet Culture Steals Your Well-Being

Kai Hibbard's body has been through a lot. Best known as the former *Biggest Loser* contestant who ended up speaking out about the show's dangerous weight-loss practices, Hibbard—now a social worker—developed seriously disordered eating behaviors during the show that took a lasting toll on her mental and physical health. In addition to losing her period and having her hair fall out in clumps during her most restrictive phase of eating, after the show ended she developed disconcerting new symptoms: severe fatigue, persistent body aches, and a scary moment when she couldn't lift her arms. Yet over the two-year period when she was trying to get help for these symptoms, every doctor she saw blamed the issues on her weight. "I would get diagnosed *fat*," Hibbard says. (Like most *Biggest Loser* contestants, Hibbard had regained weight after the show ended; not only does dieting not work long-term for practically anyone, but contestants on that particular reality show seem to have gone through some especially profound metabolic changes thanks to the extreme starvation they endured.[1]) Hibbard's worst experience with doctors during that period came when an endocrinologist took one look at her and said, " 'So how are you managing your diabetes?' " she recalls. "I don't have diabetes. I've never had diabetes—my blood sugars throughout my entire life have been perfect. She just looked at my body and assumed that that's why I was there."

What Hibbard had, it turns out, was rheumatoid arthritis (RA), an autoimmune disorder that causes the body to attack its own joints and other tissues. It's a progressive disease that, left untreated, can cause lasting harm to various parts of the body. "I'm pretty pissed off because RA can damage your internal organs, and I spent two years where possibly my body was attacking itself," she says. "It may have shortened my life span because they were so biased about my weight."

Unfortunately, Kai Hibbard is not alone. Millions of people in larger bodies have walked into doctors' offices and been "diagnosed" on sight with a host of ailments they don't have, or told to lose weight to treat something that instead requires real, evidence-based medicine. Ragen Chastain, the health coach we heard from in Chapter 3, once went to the doctor for *strep throat* and was told to lose weight, as if somehow weight loss could cure an acute infection. (It can't.) Chastain pushed to get the antibiotics she needed, but many people aren't as comfortable standing up to health-care providers as she and Hibbard are. Doctors are authority figures, and it can be intimidating to disagree with them—no matter your size. In our weight-obsessed health-care environment, it's all too easy for genuine ailments to go undiagnosed, compromising people's health and shortening their lives, all because of their doctors' biased ideas about body size.

The Weight of Stigma

There's no question that a *correlation* exists between higher BMI and negative health outcomes such as diabetes, heart disease, and some forms of cancer. (That is, most research shows that people in larger bodies have a higher risk of getting those diseases.) The question is *why*—and that's where diet culture leads us astray.

Diet culture's conventional wisdom is that this correlation

exists because living in a larger body *causes* health problems—like, hello, *everybody knows* that being fat is bad for your health. Yet as discussed earlier, the one golden rule in statistics is that *correlation does not equal causation:* if there's a correlation between variables A and B, we can never say that variable A *causes* variable B unless we've controlled for every possible factor that could be the real cause of variable B. In weight science, we can't say that being in a larger body *causes* poor health, because we haven't controlled for some very important confounding variables. Research shows that experiencing weight stigma—aka weight bias, weight-based discrimination, fatphobia, or all the stereotypes that diet culture feeds us about larger bodies—is one of those confounding variables, and it's a doozy.

Weight stigma has been linked to an increased risk of mental-health conditions such as disordered eating, emotional distress, negative body image, low self-esteem, and depression.[2] That's understandable—it feels awful to be stigmatized, and people in larger bodies get stigma from all sides. They're often bullied and shamed in school, at home, walking down the street, and in the doctor's office. They're subjected to harmful stereotypes about their character because of their body size—stereotypes I won't repeat here because they're not even remotely true, and I don't want to give them any more airtime than they already get in diet culture. Because of the pervasive weight bias in our society, people in larger bodies are less likely to get hired for jobs—and even when they do, they're paid lower wages than their thin peers.[3] They're also constantly barraged with media messages about the so-called "obesity epidemic" and the supposed perils of higher weights, which only reinforces the message they've already gotten from all corners of society that their bodies are a problem to be solved. Anyone who has experienced this steady drip of negativity about an aspect of their appearance can tell you it's a recipe for feeling like shit about yourself.

What you may not know is that abundant scientific evidence

shows that weight stigma is also an independent risk factor for an array of negative *physical*-health outcomes, such as diabetes and heart disease, regardless of people's actual body size.[4] That means two people at the same point on the BMI chart can have very different physical-health risks depending on the degree of weight stigma they've experienced and internalized in their life. A person in a smaller body with a lot of weight-based self-loathing may actually be at *greater* risk for poor health outcomes than a person in a much larger body who's learned to accept their size and fight back against weight stigma. (That's quite a feat for anyone living in diet culture, but it can be done, as we'll discuss in Part II.)

Weight stigma can contribute to health problems in a number of ways. Perhaps the most obvious one is that it's stressful to be stigmatized for your size, and stress takes a physical toll on your body. The scientific term for this toll is *allostatic load,* meaning the cumulative effect of chronic stressors on multiple systems in the body: the cardiovascular system, the sympathetic and parasympathetic nervous systems, and metabolism. Because it looks at the entire body rather than isolated parts, allostatic load has been shown to be a more robust predictor of chronic-disease risk than other markers. And the research is clear that weight stigma has seriously detrimental whole-body effects. One study that followed close to 1,000 participants for ten years found that those who reported experiencing significant weight stigma over that period were twice as likely to have a high allostatic load as those who didn't — regardless of actual BMI.[5] In other words, weight stigma is an *independent* risk factor for physiological stress.

What's more, the researchers in this study found that the health risks posed by weight stigma are greater than what the researchers called "poor-quality dietary patterns" — in diet culture's terms, eating "bad" foods. I repeat: *Weight stigma has been shown to pose a greater risk to your health than what you eat.* Diet culture's new avatar, the Wellness Diet, is forever going on about how food can make or break your health, but the evidence indicates that food has less bearing on disease risk than weight-based discrimination does. It really makes you think twice about all those public-health initiatives that shame people for their size under the guise of getting them to eat "healthier" food.

Even seemingly subtle forms of weight stigma have been shown to cause physiological stress. In 2015 researchers at UCLA conducted a laboratory experiment that exposed a group of young women to a weight-stigmatizing intervention: the participants were told they would not be allowed to participate in a group shopping activity with designer clothing because their size and shape "aren't ideal" (the implication being they might stretch or rip the clothes if they tried them on).[6] The researchers measured the participants' levels of the stress hormone cortisol before and after the intervention; when people were exposed to weight stigma, they found, their cortisol levels increased.

Intriguingly, for people who already perceived themselves as "heavy," those levels remained elevated for the duration of the experiment—their bodies stayed in a stressed-out state well after the stigmatizing incident was over. The participants who saw themselves as "average" weight, by contrast, returned to their baseline cortisol levels quickly after exposure to the weight stigma. And self-perception didn't line up with actual body size: 50 percent of the women who self-identified as "heavy" were in the "normal" BMI category, while a handful of those who identified as "average" were in the "overweight" or "obese" category. (These numbers are understandable, given that diet culture leads most women to see themselves as "too big" and makes it difficult for people in larger bodies to feel they don't need to shrink themselves.)

This squares with other research showing that body *image* is a much stronger predictor of health than body size. A 2008 study of a representative sample of the U.S. population—more than 170,000 people of all races, education levels, and ages—looked at how participants' body image related to their health.[7] The larger the difference between someone's current weight and their perceived "ideal" weight, the researchers found, the more mental- and physical-health problems they'd had in the past month—regardless of their actual BMI. The effect was stronger in women than in men, but the pattern held true across the board. That means two people of the exact same size could have wildly different health outcomes depending solely on their degree of body acceptance. Wanting to shrink your body means poorer health, no matter your size.

What's more, experiencing weight stigma has been shown to increase people's likelihood of weight *gain* and decrease their chances of weight loss. There's nothing wrong with weight gain or being in a larger body, and you'll never find me applauding weight loss (I'll leave that to diet culture, which does more than enough applauding for all of us combined). But you deserve to know the truth about what diet culture is selling you. In this case, diet culture makes weight stigma out to be "motivation" for people to lose weight, but in fact there's evidence that it does quite the opposite. A large-scale study published in 2013, for example, found that people who experienced discrimination based on their size were about two and a half times more likely to have moved into the "obese" category on the BMI chart within four years than folks who did not experience such discrimination.[8] Those effects held true when controlling for age, sex, ethnicity, education, and baseline BMI—meaning that regardless of their starting size, people who experienced more weight stigma were more likely to gain weight over the long run. Another large-scale study from 2017 found that people who experience weight-based discrimination have almost 60 percent greater odds of being physically inactive than those who do not experience it—again, independent of BMI.[9] And numerous studies have shown that when people are exposed to weight stigma in experimental settings, it leads them to eat *more,* not less.[10] So much for stigma as incentive to restrict food intake.

There are numerous reasons why people react in these ways when stigmatized for their weight. One is that they tend to avoid putting themselves in situations where discrimination is likely. Often that means avoiding physical activity, because gyms are typically hotbeds of diet culture, and moving your body in an outdoor setting can invite negative comments from strangers. Many people also have internalized messages from diet culture telling them that larger bodies are incapable of movement. "I limited myself from some activities, especially physical ones, because I thought that maybe my body wouldn't be able to do it," says Aaron Flores, now a dietitian specializing in Health At Every Size® and a Certified Body Trust® provider, who grew up in a somewhat larger body and then gained weight in college. "As my body was getting larger, I became less trusting of my body and what it could do," he says. (As we'll discuss in Chapter 10, there are many things you can do to increase your physical capacities at *any* size.)

Meanwhile, we don't know exactly why people tend to eat more when they're made to feel stigmatized for their size. One reason may be "last-supper mentality," where people who anticipate going on a diet tomorrow feel they need to eat as much as they can today. As I've seen in my clients (and as I experienced myself in my disordered-eating days), the "diet starts tomorrow" mind-set almost inevitably leads to increased eating, and even to bingeing—particularly on foods that are likely to be labeled "off-limits" once the diet begins.

Institutional Fatphobia

People of all sizes can be stigmatized for their size, but people in larger bodies generally experience higher levels of weight stigma than those in smaller bodies. As activist and author Virgie Tovar explains, there are three levels of fatphobia: the intrapersonal (within-person) level, the interpersonal (between-people) level, and the institutional level.[11] The first is all about how fatphobia affects an individual's self-image, and that's the kind of internalized weight stigma that the vast majority of people in this culture have experienced, regardless of their actual size. The fact that we pretty much all have some level of intrapersonal weight stigma in our society is one of the hallmarks of living in diet culture.

The second level, the interpersonal, is about how other people perceive you and treat you. People in smaller bodies may experience fatphobia on this level when someone in their life foists their own disordered views on them, which sadly often happens when a parent or caregiver has an untreated eating disorder or body dysmorphia that makes them see their child as unacceptably large. For the most part, though, people in larger bodies are the ones who bear the brunt of fatphobia at the interpersonal level.

The third level, institutional fatphobia, exclusively affects people in larger bodies. When physical spaces such as airplane seats and restaurant booths fail to accommodate you, or when you can't find clothes large enough to fit you at mainstream stores, or when people your size are represented in the media only as hurtful stereotypes, that's institutional fatphobia.

Lack of access to quality medical care — recall Kai Hibbard's misdiagnosis at the beginning of this chapter — is another form of institutional fatphobia, and it is rampant. Folks in larger bodies often are stigmatized for their size at the doctor's office, experiencing explicit as well as implicit bias from physicians, nurses, dietitians, and other health-care professionals.[12] This bias can come in the form of endorsing harmful, diet culture–driven beliefs that people in larger bodies are undisciplined and unwilling to follow health recommendations, which in turn affects the interaction between provider and patient. Or implicit bias might manifest itself in the provider's speaking more curtly and with less empathy to patients in larger bodies than to patients in smaller ones. Primary-care providers generally also spend less time with their larger-bodied patients, and they are likelier to rate those encounters as a waste of time. (This particular detail breaks my heart; helping my clients in larger bodies recover from diet culture—and getting to witness their insight, resilience, and self-compassion in that process—has been an incredibly rewarding and meaningful way to spend my time.)

Weight stigma from health-care providers can be subtle, but people pick up on it—especially those who've experienced a lot of stigma in their lives and are highly attuned to it. A typical visit to the doctor has a number of moments reminding patients what they experience all the time in diet culture: that larger bodies are devalued and smaller ones are privileged. Weighing a person, asking what they eat or how much physical activity they get, and giving unsolicited weight-loss advice are all moments when a doctor's or nurse's implicit weight bias can shine through. Meanwhile, the simple physical design and accessibility of the space can add to the stigma that people feel at health-care facilities: waiting-room chairs that are too small, blood-pressure cuffs that don't fit, and examination gowns that don't fully cover the body. All of these can induce feelings of shame and humiliation, even if the provider exhibits no overt signs of weight bias.

Experiencing this kind of institutional fatphobia at the doctor's office has a demonstrable impact on people's health. For one thing, it causes them to delay or skip medical visits, which can lead to poorer health outcomes down the line.[13] Rates of cervical cancer, for example, are higher among higher-weight people not because of their size but because weight stigma makes them more apt to avoid routine medical care such as Pap smears. (In some cases, it makes doctors unwilling even to *perform* Pap smears.) As a result, cervical abnormalities go undetected for longer than they would in smaller-bodied patients.[14]

People in larger bodies are also often prescribed weight loss rather than being given necessary testing and treatment, which can have disastrous consequences. A young woman named Rebecca Hiles, for example, had lung cancer that went undiagnosed for more than six years because doctors blamed her persistent cough and shortness of breath on her weight, failing to run the appropriate tests.[15] By the time Hiles got diagnosed, half of her left lung was black and rotting, and the organ had to be removed. Her surgeon told her that getting the proper diagnosis five years sooner could've saved her lung.

In general, research shows that people in larger bodies may not receive medical care until their conditions are more advanced, and therefore more difficult to treat. Health-care professionals then blame the severity of the condition on the person's weight, thereby exacerbating weight stigma. Moreover, when people do finally bite the bullet and seek out medical care, they may be so stressed by the stigma they encounter—or simply by memories of past stigma experienced in doctors' offices—that they can't give the provider's advice their full attention, or discount that advice because it's coming from someone who devalues them.

Maria Grazia, a participant in my online course on intuitive eating who's lived in a larger body her whole life, has felt stigmatized by physicians since the age of eight, when she went to the doctor after a terrible bout of German measles prevented her from holding down any food or water for several days. "I thought I was dying," she says, "and what does [the doctor] say to me? 'Oh wow, look at you, it looks like you've lost weight. That's great!' I felt like I was dying, and he's congratulating me on losing weight!"

Internal-medicine physician Jennifer Gaudiani sees the overwhelming evidence of weight stigma in her field and doesn't hold back: "Doctors keep touting this so-called 'obesity epi-demic,' and as with so many systems of oppression, I'm pretty convinced we're the ones who caused it." By focusing on weight and telling people to shrink their bodies, physicians stigmatize people in a way that does real harm.

It's time for a change. "We have to stop doing what we've been doing and take some responsibility," Gaudiani says.

A Vicious Cycle

Because of this pervasive cultural stigma, larger-bodied people are more likely to have tried to lose weight than their smaller-bodied counterparts. Yet attempts at intentional weight loss don't work in the long run, as we've discussed. Instead, these attempts most often lead to *weight cycling*—the yo-yo of weight loss and regain that's all too familiar to most dieters—which, it turns out, is also bad for your health.

Weight cycling has been associated with an increased risk of cardiovascular problems and higher mortality from all causes. Indeed, some research indicates that weight cycling can account for *all* of the excess mortality risks for certain diseases associated with being in a larger body.[16] One large-scale, long-term study followed more than 3,100 people over thirty-two years; it found weight cycling correlated with an increased risk of death from all causes and an increased risk of developing coronary heart disease, even after controlling for BMI and other potential confounding factors such as preexisting illness and smoking.[17] Not only that, but the relative risks attributable to weight cycling were comparable to the risks that typically get blamed on being in a larger body—suggesting that if *all* studies were to control for weight cycling, any excess risk from so-called "over-weight" or "obesity" might disappear.

Another large-scale study, which followed a nationally representative group of nearly 8,500 U.S. adults and took weight measurements at five different points in time, likewise linked weight fluctuation with an increased risk of death from all causes and death from cardiovascular disease—again independent of BMI, preexisting illness, race, or smoking status.[18] And one of the biggest studies I've seen, which followed more than 6.7 million participants in South Korea, found that those with the greatest degree of weight cycling had a 53 percent higher risk of death from all causes, and a 14 percent greater risk of heart attack and stroke, than those whose weight stayed stable—no matter their body size.[19]

The reasons for the association between weight cycling and poor health outcomes are still being investigated. One likely explanation is that weight cycling leads to fluctuations in blood pressure, heart rate, nervous-system activity, kidney-filtration rate, blood sugar, and blood lipids—all known cardiovascular risk factors.[20] The swings in these variables put an extra strain on the heart and may damage the kidneys and blood vessels, which in turn increases the toll on the cardiovascular system. One study of more than 12,400 adults showed that for people in the "obese" BMI category, weight cycling and short-term weight loss were strong predictors of developing high blood pressure within about two years.[21] Another study found that women in the "obese" BMI category who had weight-cycled were significantly more likely to have high blood pressure than those who hadn't.[22] Weight cycling has also been associated with increased metabolic and cardiovascular risk factors among people in the "normal-weight" BMI category.[23] When a person's weight stays stable over time, by contrast, that individual generally does not experience the same kinds of fluctuations in blood pressure or other cardiovascular risk factors. (This holds true for people in bodies of all sizes.)

Until all research can control for weight cycling and weight stigma, we can't say that being at the higher end of the BMI spectrum *causes* any health conditions—even if higher weights are *associated* with these health conditions. Remember that statistical golden rule: Correlation does not equal causation. Moreover, even if weight *did* have some causal effect on people's health (which is possible—but again, we can't know until we control for weight stigma and weight cycling), we don't have a known way for more than a tiny fraction of people to lose weight and keep it off permanently.

The long-term "success" rate of intentional weight-loss efforts is in the single digits, by most researchers' accounts. For the overwhelming majority of people, therefore, intentional weight loss is going to result only in weight cycling. As neuroscientist and author Sandra Aamodt puts it, "Almost all dieting is yo-yo dieting."[24] And from all the research we've just discussed, we know that yo-yo dieting negatively affects people's health. So it truly is a vicious cycle: people pursue weight loss in a bid to improve their health, only to put it at greater risk; then, if they develop health problems, they're told to lose weight to cure them.

And so the cycle continues.

Disordered Eating and Your Health

As a child, Virgie Tovar remembers having a blissful phase of body acceptance that lasted through preschool. By kindergarten, though, she had already absorbed the message that her body was too big and needed to be made smaller, stat. For the rest of her childhood, she wanted nothing more than to be thin.

Tovar started dieting in elementary school. Every summer she would restrict her eating even more severely, hoping to return to school transformed. It never happened. She kept trying, though, using increasingly disordered behaviors that, in a person who had started out thin, might have resulted in a swift diagnosis of anorexia. Because she never got thin, however, that never happened. Tovar's disordered eating continued through high school and into college—when, at age eighteen, she had an opportunity to do a short-term study-abroad program in Italy. "My fantasy was that of dieters all over," she recalls, "which is 'I'm going to go to Italy and I'm going to lose weight, and then when I come back and I'm exiting the international terminal I'm going to walk right past my family and they're not even going to recognize me.'"

Trying to make that fantasy a reality, Tovar embarked on the most restrictive diet of her life—a starvation regimen, really. Her body was not a fan. "Nearing the end of the trip I began to have really intense dizzy spells, such that I could only stand for about five to ten minutes in any stretch, and then I would be exhausted and have to lie down," Tovar says. One evening that happened while she was out by herself in the downtown area of the city where she was staying. "I got so dizzy and exhausted that I lay down on a bench and fell asleep there, and I woke up at three a.m.," she says. "Out in public, on a bench. And I just think to myself, *This is the road that diet culture takes us on—and to deny how sinister it is, is to deny the truth.*"

That's Tovar's perspective now, as a writer and activist who speaks out about the dangers of diet culture and fatphobia, but at the time she couldn't see it. Even though she knew she was putting herself at risk by eating so restrictively, she says, "that didn't stop me. I didn't understand the connection between starvation and what was happening to me. I just thought it was this weirdly coincidental thing."

Disordered eating jeopardizes your health and safety in major ways like that. Severely restricting your food intake as Tovar did puts you at risk—not only of passing out, but also of liver damage, osteoporosis, heart attacks, and death. Purging carries many of the same risks, and it can cause additional cardiac problems such as palpitations, arrhythmias, and heart failure, in addition to painful tearing of the esophagus and an increased risk of esophageal cancer. Laxative abuse can cause electrolyte imbalances and severe dehydration. And many people with disordered eating, as well as those with compulsive exercise behaviors, experience hormonal abnormalities, among them irregular or missing periods, low sex drive, infertility, and thyroid problems.

Disordered eating and compulsive exercise can also trigger IBS and other digestive issues and functional gut disorders, as we discussed in Chapter 3. Bingeing, restricting, purging, and other disordered behaviors can cause gas, bloating, constipation, and diarrhea. Some people who engage in disordered-eating behaviors also experience gastritis—a painful inflammation of the stomach lining—and acid reflux. And all that's to say nothing of the headaches, fatigue, "brain fog," and general malaise that disordered eating and overexercise can cause.

Diet culture's new guise, the Wellness Diet, encourages people to blame food for these issues—to search for hidden "intolerances" and eliminate long lists of foods from their lives, under the assumption that this will fix their digestion and overall health. Yet I've seen far too many people who went down this rabbit hole, only to end up exacerbating both their underlying disordered eating and their digestive issues: the real problem wasn't *what* they were eating but *how*.

I had a client I saw a few times for nutrition counseling— let's call her Megan. (All of my clients' names and identifying details have been changed to protect their privacy.) During our intake appointment, Megan reported that she'd been having recurring digestive problems for the past year or so, and that she'd seen a bevy of doctors—all of whom told her to cut out various foods. One advised her to limit gluten at first, but when she tested negative for celiac disease he switched to recommending a low-FODMAP diet. Another doctor instructed her to cut out dairy. Yet another one diagnosed her with small intestinal bacterial overgrowth (SIBO) and put her on an antibiotic, which didn't seem to help much.

None of the doctors had asked Megan about her relationship with food or screened her for disordered eating. But when we started to talk about her behaviors with food, I quickly saw what was going on: a devotee of "clean eating" who was struggling with orthorexia, she ate meals that consisted primarily—sometimes entirely—of vegetables. For most of the day, her snacks were nothing but fruits, vegetables, and other "whole" foods, which meant she was consuming an obscene amount of fiber—a well-known cause of bloating, gas, and other intestinal woes that often get blamed on "intolerances." (Fiber in food is usually thought of as a beneficial thing; as cases like Megan's reveal, however, it's possible to overdo it.) Not only that, but the deprivation of eating so "clean" (and so little food of any real *substance*) usually got to be so intense by the end of Megan's day that she wound up bingeing on whatever snack foods she kept in the house. Most were supposedly "healthy" options that contained—you guessed it—lots of added fiber.

Orthorexia pretends to be all about health and wellness. It can actually be extremely harmful to your health. Another client of mine, whom I'll call Jean, landed in the ER several times because her sodium levels were dangerously low. She thought that drinking water and avoiding salty foods were "healthy" behaviors, and she did them so obsessively that she wound up basically drowning her body, putting herself at risk of seizures, coma, and death. Like quite a few orthorexia clients I've known, Jean had also cut so many foods from her diet that she was literally starving; in many cases orthorexia can morph into anorexia, which is why the line between them is so blurry.

For folks in this boat, the attempt at "healthy eating" may start out having little to do with weight, but eventually their bodies can dip dangerously below their weight set range—even if they're still in larger bodies and never become emaciated. At that point, their bodies actually start consuming themselves in order to stay alive. This was evident in Jean's blood work, which suggested that her liver was essentially eating itself because her food was not furnishing enough energy.[25] Even if they never reach such an acute level of starvation, people with orthorexia can suffer from vitamin and mineral deficiencies—as well as excesses. Katie Dalebout, whom we heard from in Chapter 4, got a calcium kidney stone likely because her intake of calcium from her "clean-eating" diet was so high. "I know that that wouldn't have happened other than from my orthorexia," Dalebout says. "There's no family history. It's very rare for women to get them in general, especially young women."

You don't need an eating-disorder diagnosis to suffer serious health effects from disordered eating. In fact, weight bias plays a role in the diagnosing of eating disorders. Too many medical and mental-health providers still hold an outdated belief that the only way to have an eating disorder is if you look emaciated or are "underweight" on the BMI chart. But make no mistake: the harmful effects of disordered-eating behaviors such as restrictive eating and purging are just as real for people in larger bodies as for those in smaller ones. "My anorexia was not worse when I was in a smaller body than it was when I was in a larger body," says Rachel Millner, now a psychologist specializing in eating disorders, who struggled with anorexia when she was in graduate school. "People's reactions to it were different, but the anorexia wasn't worse—I was doing the exact same things at a lower weight as I was at a higher weight." Yet weight bias kept anyone from recognizing the disordered behaviors when Millner's body was larger.

Some people don't get diagnosed until after the fact, if they do at all. Kristy Fassio, a personal trainer who now also works in the mental-health field helping people recover from disordered eating, remembers a session with a new therapist that blew her mind. "She was giving me this intake, and she goes, 'OK, so that was your anorexic period,' and I was like, 'I'm sorry, what now?'" Fassio says. "It clearly was, but [I thought] *I wasn't tiny, so how could I have had an eating disorder?*"

I've always lived in a smaller body, yet weight bias kept me too from being diagnosed when I was in the depths of my disorder. When I mentioned my disordered-eating behaviors to my therapist at the time and told her some of my loved ones were concerned I might have an eating disorder, she said that couldn't possibly be the case—I wasn't thin enough. She used the phrase *You're not a slight person,* which says a lot about how subjective the process of diagnosing an eating disorder can be. It also shows how many clinicians, caught up in looking for what they imagine to be physical signs that someone is struggling, miss the bigger picture: you can't tell from the outside whether someone is engaging in disordered eating.

Surgical Scars

Weight-loss surgery—aka bariatric surgery—is often touted as the answer to weight cycling. If dieting doesn't work, the reasoning goes, why not cut out or constrict people's stomachs so that they physically *can't* eat as much? Surely that's a permanent solution for weight loss and health, right? Erm, no. As nutrition professor and weight-science expert Lindo Bacon puts it, "Bariatric surgery... would be more appropriately labeled high-risk, disease-inducing cosmetic surgery than a health-enhancing procedure."[26] Despite all the marketing—by surgeons and health-care facilities that, remember, stand to make tens of thousands of dollars for each of these procedures they perform—weight-loss surgery is more of a life-stealing intervention than a lifesaving one, for many reasons.

Bariatric surgery can take several forms, each with its own set of potential complications. Granted, virtually all surgeries carry some level of risk, and the mere act of undergoing surgery can potentially be harmful. But there are particular risks to altering the digestive system. The most seemingly benign of these alterations is lap-band surgery (aka the laparoscopic band), which Linda Aubuchon opted for in Chapter 4. In this surgery, a band with an inflatable balloon is placed around the stomach; the tightness of the band can then be adjusted by adding saline to the balloon, restricting the size of the stomach. Lap-band surgery is generally considered less invasive than the other forms, but it still carries some pretty major risks.

Take Sarah Harry's experience, for instance. Harry is now a body-positive mental-health counselor and yoga teacher in Australia, but two decades ago she was just a young woman in a larger body, desperate to lose weight. She had recovered from bulimia not long before, but her body image still wasn't fully healed—so she decided to have lap-band surgery. "Pretty much from day one I was in chronic pain and vomiting," she says, which made her feel like she was regressing in her recovery from the eating disorder. But it was when she had the band adjusted that things got really scary. "They filled it up with saline, and they filled it up to the top so I couldn't even swallow my saliva," she says. When she called the doctor's office to let them know what was happening, "they went into a panic," she says. "I had to be admitted to the hospital because you'll die if that happens. You have a very short amount of time actually if you can't swallow. I didn't know that 'til the doctor told me."

Other adjustments were hardly any better. "A couple of times they did it too tight and I could only swallow tiny, tiny bits of water, which of course put me into the hospital again," she says. The chronic pain also remained. Then, as lap bands sometimes do, Harry's slipped out of position within the first year, which caused her to wake up choking in the middle of the night. The doctors told her she had to have a second surgery to get it fixed, so she did—and the problems were exactly the same. Eventually, like Aubuchon, Harry had all the saline taken out of the band so that it stopped constricting her stomach. All in all, as she experienced, the lap band was anything but the low-impact intervention it was made out to be.

Of course, not everyone who has one of these surgeries will have major problems like Harry did. I know some people reading this—maybe even you—might've had relatively positive experiences with the lap band or other forms of bariatric surgery. I'm genuinely glad you're doing well, and I don't want to discount the experience of anyone who feels they've benefited from this kind of procedure.

What I'm saying, though, is that if you haven't had one of these surgeries, I don't recommend getting one. The potential for harm is too great to roll the dice, and it's unclear if there are any real benefits. I understand and empathize with the desire to escape weight stigma through surgery (or dieting, or any other means), because the effects of stigma are real and harmful. But bariatric surgery and weight-loss efforts pose significant risks to your overall health and well-being, and there is no proven long-term way to shrink people's bodies, including by surgical alteration.

Consider the surgeries that remove part or most of the stomach. The gastric sleeve, aka the sleeve gastrectomy, involves cutting out a large chunk of the stomach and sewing the remaining part into a tube shaped like a tiny shirtsleeve. Then there's the Roux-en-Y gastric bypass, which involves amputating most of the stomach, leaving only a small pouch, and bypassing most of the small intestine so that fewer nutrients are absorbed. And finally the duodenal switch is basically a combination of the first two surgeries: the stomach is cut into a sleeve, and most of the small intestine is bypassed.

Bariatric surgeries are classified as restrictive, malabsorptive, or both. The lap band and the sleeve are considered restrictive surgeries, whereas the gastric bypass and duodenal switch are both restrictive and malabsorptive. If those categories sound like forms of disordered eating or disease, it's because they basically are: restrictive surgeries "work" by restricting the amount of food people can eat to a minuscule amount (on the order of what I've seen in clients with active anorexia), and malabsorptive surgeries "work" by causing reduced digestion and absorption of nutrients, including calories, protein, fat, and essential vitamins and minerals. Both classes of weight-loss surgery force the body to consume or absorb less food, in the hope of permanently shrinking it. (Notice I said *hope;* more on that shortly.)

Some of the most common nutritional complications after malabsorptive surgeries are deficiencies in protein, vitamin B-12, vitamin D, calcium, and iron. Because these particular deficiencies are relatively well-known, most bariatric providers monitor patients for them and recommend nutritional supplements. Yet patients' adherence to these recommendations is decidedly mixed.[27] After bariatric surgery, people typically need special vitamin and mineral supplements that can cost as much as $125 per month, because standard multivitamins don't suffice. Many patients don't know the nuances of what they're supposed to be taking, or can't afford the special vitamins and take regular multis instead. I've even heard of some adults taking kids' chewable vitamins, which are definitely not enough for someone with malabsorption issues. Even more disturbing, many health-care providers don't realize their post-bariatric-surgery patients are at risk of additional deficiencies in nutrients including vitamins A and K, other B vitamins, zinc, copper, and essential fats. Providers' monitoring and prevention of these deficiencies—which can lead to terrible (and sometimes irreversible) consequences for the immune, nervous, and muscular systems—are woefully inadequate.

Another common complication, dumping syndrome, is about as appealing as it sounds. After a person eats, the contents of the stomach empty too quickly (or "dump") into the small intestine.

Dumping syndrome can affect people who've had either restrictive or malabsorptive surgeries,[28] and the symptoms include nausea, vomiting, abdominal pain and cramping, diarrhea, bloating, extreme fullness, sweating, weakness, dizziness, flushing, rapid or irregular heartbeat, and low blood sugar. Nutrient deficiencies are generally more dangerous, but dumping syndrome is a lot more uncomfortable—not to mention potentially embarrassing—on a day-to-day basis. Dumping syndrome can also exacerbate or bring about new deficiencies, given that vomiting results in a dangerous loss of nutrients, and having uncomfortable GI symptoms can lead to the avoidance of important food groups. Dumping syndrome isn't a temporary thing, either; it can last the rest of your life. I've seen clients with symptoms of it more than ten years after their bariatric surgery.

Bariatric surgery—particularly gastric bypass—may also trigger the onset of addiction and substance-use disorders. A number of studies have shown that alcohol-use disorder and illicit-drug use are significantly higher in patients who've had Roux-en-Y gastric bypass surgery a few years before.[29] The risk is higher in younger men who already drank some alcohol (as opposed to those who drank none), but one large study found that the prevalence of alcohol-use disorder for patients of all ages and genders more than *doubled* by seven years after surgery.[30] In that study, 20 percent of people who hadn't had any issues with alcohol in the year before bariatric surgery reported alcohol abuse at some point within five years after having gastric bypass.

Some have hypothesized this is because of "transfer addiction," where people once "addicted to food" switched to alternate substances now that they couldn't eat as much. But "food addiction" isn't a real thing—even though you might *feel* addicted to certain foods—and when people experience addiction-like patterns in their eating, it's actually a symptom of restriction and deprivation, not true addiction.[31] Instead, the incidence of substance abuse after bariatric surgery is thought to be due to the physiological changes that occur with surgery, which make people more sensitive to the effects of substances than they were before.[32] Alcohol, for example, is absorbed faster, reaches higher levels in the body, and takes longer to clear from the bloodstream after gastric bypass. These physiological changes cause alcohol to hit the brain much more quickly than it did before, resulting in a much higher high. "What you see for folks who've had the surgery is more of a sharp high that's similar to what people experience with cocaine," says psychotherapist Lisa DuBreuil, who specializes in addictions and eating disorders. And when we experience a high like that, we're more likely to get addicted. "Substances that hit the brain more quickly are more addictive," she explains. The research to date has focused primarily on gastric bypass, but DuBreuil says she's been seeing clinically that people with the gastric sleeve are having similar experiences with alcohol.

However, the most serious potential complication of bariatric surgery is death. A large-scale 2005 study looked at mortality rates for more than 16,000 people who had bariatric surgery and found that 4.6 percent of them had died a year after surgery.[33] Other estimates are more conservative, and recent surgical advances may have led to a reduction in the risk of death. Still, one of those conservative estimates shows that within thirty days of having bariatric surgery, 3 out of every 1,000 patients die.[34] That's the same percentage of people who die of anaphylactic shock in the U.S.[35] I don't know about you, but those numbers don't make me want to start playing fast and loose with severe allergic reactions.

The most recent review of the evidence shows that people who've had bariatric surgery have a significantly higher risk of death than the general population, as well as a risk of suicide that's up to 8.7 times greater in women (and 5.5 times greater in men) than people who haven't had bariatric surgery.[36] Research is mixed on whether people who've had bariatric surgery have a significantly different risk of mortality than control groups made up of people in the "obese" BMI category; some studies show a reduced risk for folks who've had the surgery. But many of the latter findings may be flawed, as one 2011 study pointed out, because the control groups in those trials had confounding factors such as preexisting disease diagnoses, racial differences, and other characteristics that could explain their higher mortality rates.[37] In other words, the control groups may have had a higher risk of death than the bariatric surgery groups *even before surgery*, rendering the comparisons essentially meaningless. And the survival differences between the bariatric-surgery groups and the control groups in most of those studies were modest at best, so any benefits from surgery might have decreased or disappeared if the researchers had accounted for confounding variables.

By the way, you know how weight-loss surgery is touted as a permanent way to lose weight? Yeah, not so much: The majority of people who have bariatric surgery regain some or all of the weight they lost.[38] And just as with dieting, the likelihood of regaining weight increases over time: two years after surgery, 46 percent of patients have had significant weight regain; by four years post-surgery that number jumps to more than 63 percent, and likely continues to grow as the years go on. That's something you probably won't hear in a bariatric consultation. Weight-loss surgery is usually billed as pretty foolproof — the answer for anyone (or anyone in a "large enough" body to qualify for the procedure) who's had trouble losing weight and keeping it off through traditional dieting. This surgery will fix you forever! you're told. You can't go wrong, because your stomach won't allow it! Then, if you do regain weight, you're made to feel like *you're* the problem — just as in all other forms of diet culture. Rest assured, though: if you happen to be one of those people who's regained weight after bariatric surgery, it's not because you're some weirdo; it's actually very common.

What About Physical Discomfort?

By now I hope you understand that most chronic diseases blamed on weight can most likely be explained by other phenomena, such as weight stigma and weight cycling. (And that correlation does not equal causation.) But what about conditions such as joint pain or difficulty with movement? Those *have* to be caused by higher weight, right?

Not necessarily.

"I think one of the big problems with a society that's so ready to credit thinness with anything good and to blame fatness for anything bad is that we get this idea that the only way to improve anything is by somehow making our bodies smaller," health coach Ragen Chastain says. "And so it gives people the idea that there's nothing to do except lose weight, when in fact there are many, many things that we can do to improve mobility, to improve flexibility." Moreover, she says, "building strength is something that works at all sizes, whereas weight loss is something that works for almost no one. If you think your current body size is the problem, dieting gives you a 66 percent chance to make that 'problem' a bigger problem." It simply is not evidence-based medicine to say that people "need to lose weight" for any health reasons, because *we have no safe, sustainable method of producing weight loss.*

If weight stigma and weight cycling were out of the picture, it's possible that body size could still be a risk factor for some health issues. But *we just don't know*—because controlling for those two things would be a tall order in our society at this point in time. "You cannot study fat people in this culture without also studying a history of dieting, without also studying a history of stigma," Chastain says. Speaking of tall orders, she points out that being tall is a risk factor for certain health conditions.

Male-pattern baldness is another risk factor, as mentioned earlier. Whatever your ethnic background is, it almost certainly puts you at higher risk of one health condition or another—because of racism, genetics, or both. Having light skin generally makes you less susceptible to the first, but it raises your risk of skin cancer. Yet with every condition other than body size, nobody is saying we should try to change central characteristics of people's bodies in order to reduce the risk of certain health conditions. And even though weight can be temporarily suppressed, people's general weight range is a trait as genetically determined as height. So why are we telling people to change their weight?

The forms of physical discomfort that get blamed on weight—mobility issues, chafing, shortness of breath, to name a few—all have solutions that don't involve weight loss, as we'll discuss in Chapter 10. Meanwhile, weight stigma often magnifies the discomfort of these physical issues. As author and body-liberation advocate Sonya Renee Taylor explains, the concept of discomfort means different things to different people. "There's a lot of work around unpacking language like this. What does *uncomfortable* mean? Because it's a vague word," she says. For some people, it means their clothes are too tight. "Is that because you're unwilling to go up a size in the clothes you're wearing? And if so, let's talk about why that is," Taylor says. (In diet culture, that usually has to do with not wanting to perceive yourself as larger.) "A lot of times, *uncomfortable in my body* means *uncomfortable with this new size and all the conditioning that I have received about what it means to be this size now,*" she explains, and we need to work to untangle our beliefs about weight and size from ideas about what physical comfort means. "At the end of the day, usually it isn't about the weight," Taylor says. "There are markers and indicators of wellness, agility, stamina, and all of these things that are absolutely independent of weight. But we have them so tied together that when our bodies change, you just automatically assume that all of those things are a function of weight gain, and that the only way they can be navigated is by weight loss."

Here's a question Taylor suggests asking yourself to help figure out if your concerns about comfort are just about comfort, not about internalized weight stigma: If you were able to do all the things you want to do with your body (climb stairs without getting winded, stop having knee pain, and so on) and never lose a single pound, would that be OK with you? If you replied no, "then we know that we're starting to get into the realm where this is much more about the stigma of weight than it is about actual, material discomfort," Taylor says. "That's something that we do often in the realm of weight: we blame our bodies for the ways in which weight stigma and bias are baked into the entirety of our society." So instead of jumping to blame your weight for any discomfort you feel, what if you could recognize that the problem isn't your body, but how you've been made to *feel* about your body? "It's important for us to keep coming back to [the fact] that it's not about you as an individual," Taylor says. "It's about a larger system that we've all been conditioned to believe in to varying degrees."

Not only does weight stigma cause people to blame their bodies for something that's the fault of diet culture, but this stigma can worsen discomfort in physical, material ways. Consider knee pain, for example: "The problem starts at the very beginning, when fat people first have knee pain," Chastain explains. "If they got the same interventions as thin people, their knees would very likely get better, but they don't. [Instead] they're told to go out and exercise and lose weight in a way that is likely to make their knees worse," because doing cardio on an injured knee doesn't usually end well. "It goes on longer and longer, so when fat people go to get their knee surgeries they're likely in a much worse state than thin people getting knee surgery," Chastain says.

The assumption that knee pain is caused by weight rather than by alignment issues, overuse, or tendinitis—conditions that affect thin people's knees, too—makes knee problems worse. As with every other health issue we've discussed, no scientific data shows that a higher BMI *causes* knee problems; there's only evidence that it's *associated* with them.[39] Because we live in diet culture, however, health-care providers misinterpret that correlation as causation. The result: larger-bodied people get treated in ways that actively worsen their health outcomes. Weight stigma is the problem here, not weight itself.

Beyond Physical Health

Truly holistic health is about so much more than what you eat, how you exercise, or how much you weigh. Yet most of what passes for "holistic" health in diet culture is exclusively about physical health—a point that integrative physician Steven Bratman made in his 2000 book, *Health Food Junkies,* and that the health-and-wellness field seems largely to have forgotten. Cutting out foods and food groups, looking for hidden causes of inflammation and "food intolerance," trying to ward off disease and extend your life span—all of these practices prioritize the physical instead of the mental, emotional, social, and spiritual aspects of life. Even the tenets of modern-day holistic health that pretend to be about healing psychological issues are often just disguised versions of prioritizing the physical—among them the belief that eliminating certain foods will ward off depression or anxiety, or the idea that exercise can be a substitute for psychotherapy or medication.

Our mental health has a huge effect on our overall health and well-being, but we tend to forget that fact because of all the "you are what you eat" rhetoric swirling around in diet culture. The truth is that you actually *aren't* what you eat. You are so much more. By reducing us down to what we eat—and offering physical "solutions" to all of our mental and emotional problems—diet culture negates the importance of many other factors that determine our well-being. As we've seen in this chapter, our health can be negatively affected by experiences of weight stigma and weight cycling. It is also profoundly influenced by the social determinants of health—elements such as socioeconomic status, race, education, and a host of other sociocultural factors largely or entirely beyond our control.

Those social determinants contribute strongly to our mental health. They also have a great deal more to do with our physical-health outcomes than whether or not we eat the amount of kale currently prescribed by the Wellness Diet. Sure, nutrition is important in the sense that we need to have *enough* food, and a wide enough variety of foods, to keep our bodies biologically satisfied and nourished. Of course those things can play a role in our overall well-being. But as we'll discuss next, a balanced relationship with food—and a balanced life—is about so much more than what we eat or how we move our bodies.

CHAPTER 6

How Diet Culture Steals Your Happiness

At the end of his podcast, *You Made It Weird,* comedian Pete Holmes often asks guests to share the time they laughed the hardest (either in recent memory or ever).* The answer is almost invariably a you-had-to-be-there type story that doesn't make a lot of sense in the retelling, often involving a well-timed quip or a spot-on observation about something that was going on in a particular moment. Pete's story was when he was swimming with a childhood friend, and as another kid swam erratically toward them, his friend turned to him and said, "In other news, like getting away from this guy..." Mine was when my husband yelled, "Hello, bird!" to a seagull in a vaguely Eastern European accent. You really had to be there.

In fact, there's a lot of evidence that you *do* have to be there—as in being present, engaging in what's happening right now rather than thinking about other things—in order to experience not just unbridled laughter, but happiness in general. Many religious and philosophical traditions have been hip to this idea for centuries, which is why practices such as meditation exist to teach people to live in the moment and bring themselves back to the present when they mentally check out. Now we also have scientific research to back them up: In a landmark 2010

---

* I love this podcast but hesitate to recommend it because of Pete's internalized fatphobia and participation in the Wellness Diet. Listen at your own risk.

study, researchers at Harvard collected data from 2,250 adults via an iPhone app, asking the participants at random moments throughout the day to record how happy they were currently feeling, what they were currently doing (or had been doing before they got interrupted by the app), and whether they'd been thinking about anything other than what they were doing — whether their minds were wandering.[1] If they were thinking about something else, they were asked to record whether it was something pleasant, neutral, or unpleasant.

The researchers found that people were happiest when their minds weren't wandering at all, even when they were doing the least-enjoyable activities, such as commuting and housework. If they were thinking about anything other than what they were doing — even if they were thinking about something pleasant — their reported happiness was significantly lower. Granted, people who are already in a bad mood might be more likely to let their minds wander. But the researchers did a time-lag analysis and found that mind wandering was the *cause,* not just a consequence, of unhappiness. Or as the title of their published paper put it, "A Wandering Mind Is an Unhappy Mind."

Of course, many things go into happiness, presence being just one. Psychologists also define happiness as having frequent experiences of positive emotions such as joy, contentment, affection, and love; having relatively infrequent experiences of negative emotions such as sadness and loneliness; and having a sense of satisfaction, meaning, identity, and worth in your life.[2] Living in line with your values, belonging to a community, having a meaningful way to contribute to the world, feeling safe and accepted, having your basic needs met — by most accounts, all of these things are essential ingredients for happiness.

Diet culture robs people of these things. By taking us out of the moment, disconnecting us from ourselves and others, threatening our sense of safety, and depriving us of our basic needs, the Life Thief actively undermines our happiness.

Not Being There

One of the things I hear about diet culture all the time from clients, online course students, and podcast listeners is a version of this:

"My social life is nonexistent."

Or this:

"I avoid going to parties, since I know there will be lots of food and alcohol around."

Or this:

"Whenever I get invited to a wedding, I start panicking about fitting into my dress and can't enjoy myself for months."

Or this:

"I can't enjoy the food at my family's holiday meal because I'm so afraid of how it'll affect my body."

Diet culture can make people so fearful of food and anxious about losing control that they can't truly participate in their lives. It isolates them, even when they're desperate for connection. In this way the Life Thief steals people's capacity for everyday joy. It keeps them from being present in all the big and small moments of their lives — moments such as anniversary dinners, birthday parties, weddings, or just lunch with a friend on a Tuesday. It keeps them from going out and engaging with the world.

If they do participate, it keeps them from truly *being there*. It always holds a part of their minds hostage. In the darkest days of my eating disorder, I was so chronically deprived of food that I would go to parties and stand by the snack table for hours, compulsively eating and beating myself up for it. I craved human connection almost as much as I craved the carbs and calories I'd been denying myself, and I would talk to whoever came by to grab a few chips or cookies, but my heart was never really in the conversation: I was absorbed in eating the food and judging myself for it. I can still clearly remember many of the things I ate during my party binges at that time—nearly two decades ago now—but I've long since forgotten what my friends and I talked about. (Although let's be real: a lot of the time we were probably talking about food and diets.)

"When you're dieting, it's kind of like when you're on the phone with somebody and you can tell they're checking email or they're texting or doing something else," says *Intuitive Eating* coauthor Evelyn Tribole. "They're participating in the conversation, the words are correct, but you can tell there's something missing. And that's what happens when you're dieting—you're missing out on your own life and the richness and the things that renew you and make you human." That's exactly it: dieting is a giant distraction from what's happening right now. It's a constant buzzing in the back of your mind, a running to-do list you can't turn off, an uninvited commentary on everything you're putting in your mouth and how your clothes are fitting and what your next workout is going to be.

This kind of life theft is so subtle that it's hard to recognize, even though it's there in every moment, stealing your attention. This isn't about finding your calling or realizing your potential (though diet culture restricts those things, too); it's about your day-to-day human existence. Your ability to grab a spontaneous bite with a friend, enjoy a piece of cake at a birthday party, eat at a drive-through on a road trip. Your ability to rock the dance floor at a wedding. Your ability to hear a quip about a seagull and laugh your ass off—instead of being so lost in your own thoughts that the wave of joy passes you by.

Identity Theft

A friend of mine named Lindsay Kite loved swimming as a kid. Along with her identical twin sister, Lexie, she was on the swim team starting in early elementary school. The Kites were fast, strong swimmers, and they did well in their competitive meets. They felt good about their bodies because of their abilities in the pool. Swimming was a huge part of their identities. At about eight years old, though, Lindsay looked at herself in the mirror in her racing swimsuit and noticed a dimple on her left thigh. "I was only in third grade, but I remember instinctively knowing that that dimple was bad, that it was a sign that I was too big, that my body was wrong," she says. That was the start of her diet culture–induced body shame, a shame that spiraled over the years until it became all-consuming for both Lindsay and her sister. "By the time we were about fifteen years old, we both had quit swimming—and a huge part of that was because we didn't want other people looking at us in our swimming suits," Lindsay says. "Our dieting and restricting hadn't solved what we perceived to be our weight problems, so it only made sense for us to just quit swimming."

It only made sense. By diet culture's twisted logic, that's exactly what we're taught to think: if your body is a source of shame in a given activity, and you're unable to shrink your body permanently (which of course almost none of us are), then *it only makes sense* to give up that activity. Even if it's something you love, something that brings you joy and fulfillment and a sense of connection to your own body. Even if it feels like an essential part of who you are.

Too many of us have lost important aspects of our identity to the Life Thief. Whether your thing is swimming, singing, dancing, acting, skydiving, or dogsledding, it's likely you've stopped doing something you once loved—or stopped seeing it as anything more than an occasional hobby—because diet culture told you your body was "wrong." What parts of yourself have you relinquished because diet culture made you afraid to be seen? What sources of joy and fulfillment and self-worth has the Life Thief taken from you?

One common way diet culture robs us of these things is by

persuading us to renounce certain foods that bring us pleasure and connect us to our loved ones or our heritage. I've had people tell me that in their efforts to lose weight or "get healthy" they swore off the tortillas that were central to the cuisine of their country of origin; or they stopped eating rice with their home-cooked Chinese meals; or they started turning down their grandmother's made-from-scratch pie (with no legitimate medical basis for avoiding those foods — like, say, a food allergy diagnosed using validated scientific tests). They cut out these foods because diet culture had demonized them and they thought that's what they were supposed to do.

Even early in my career as a dietitian, when I was still caught up in diet culture, I could nonetheless see that cutting out such culturally important foods was sad and unnecessary. Now I also recognize that these kinds of food restrictions are ways in which diet culture disconnects people from *actual* culture, from tradition and identity. Diet culture robs us of our culinary connection to who we are and where we come from.

Not only that, but diet culture steals our sense of identity at perhaps the most fundamental level: our ability to feel at home in our bodies. For however long we're on this planet, our bodies are where we live. They're our original homes, the ones we carry with us wherever we go, from the womb to our deathbeds. Feeling connected to and at peace with them is crucial to feeling safe in the world. By making us feel self-conscious and not good enough in our bodies, diet culture disconnects us from them — and thereby makes us question our very identities, our basic worthiness as human beings. By keeping us from feeling at home in our bodies, it keeps us from feeling at home in the world at large.

Of course, many other things can make us feel disconnected from our bodies, such as illnesses, disabilities, and other health issues; physical abuse and other forms of trauma; and gender dysphoria (the experience that some transgender people have of occupying a body that doesn't match their gender identity).

All of these painful experiences in relation to the body can negatively affect people's well-being and happiness, and healing the rift between mind and body can require a lot of time and support.

In the case of diet culture, all too often that healing never happens because people don't recognize the nature of the problem. They just know they hate how they look, or how other people look at them, and want to "fix" it by losing weight. Or they know they don't feel well and assume it's because they need to eliminate certain foods, not recognizing that this approach is likely to compound their malaise. Because when diet culture makes us feel uncomfortable in our own skin, the solution to feeling better is never going to be the one that diet culture prescribes. Imagine that someone stole your identity, then offered to sell it back to you—that's what diet culture does. It steals your sense of self, then sells it back to you in the form of diets, "programs," "protocols," and "plans" that will supposedly make you feel great about yourself, but that leave you feeling only worse in the end.

For Lindsay Kite, fortunately, the story didn't end with giving up swimming at age fifteen. She (along with her sister) began studying body image in college, and the things she learned resonated deeply with her experience. They didn't change her behavior right away—she still kept reflexively saying no to beach or pool invitations. But one day soon after Lindsay's college graduation, she realized she was sick and tired of letting negative thoughts about her body hold her back. She decided to go jump in a lake—literally; she put on a swimsuit and joined her friends in the water. "I learned that I could still connect with my body and [with swimming], one of the most enjoyable things I've ever been able to do," Lindsay says. "It taught me I could continue to do that for the rest of my life, regardless of what I looked like or regardless of who was watching me swim. And it absolutely has brought me some of the happiest and most connected feelings and memories I could ever have."

Today the Kite sisters hold PhDs in the study of body image. They run a nonprofit called Beauty Redefined, which is dedicated to promoting positive body image online and in live speaking events. Both women still swim for the joy of it.

Unmet Needs

Having your basic needs met is a critical component of happiness. There are rare exceptions — people who go around beaming and saying "No worries" while living in abject poverty — but for the most part it's hard to be content and fulfilled when you lack such essentials as clean water, reliable shelter, and a sense of personal safety. The trauma of living life without these basic necessities takes its toll on people's mental health.

Of course, one of those basic needs is food. When you don't have enough to eat — when you live in constant fear of deprivation — it's hard to be content. Evolution conditioned us to be anxious and on the hunt for food when it was scarce, which helped our species survive in times of famine. We wouldn't be on this planet without that mechanism, but it still feels like garbage when you're going through it. Today food *seems* abundant in the Western world, where we have places to get a snack on practically every corner, but proximity to food doesn't matter if you can't access it. Whether that's because you can't afford it or because you're on a diet that restricts it, the experience of food deprivation is very real. It's natural to feel jangly and ill at ease when you don't have enough to eat. That's what hunger does to people.

One of the classic examples of this is the Minnesota Starvation Experiment. In the 1940s, as the end of World War II drew near, a team of researchers at the University of Minnesota, led by physiologist Ancel Keys, wanted to study the effects of starvation and refeeding on the human body in order to figure out how to provide effective food aid to war-torn countries.[3] Finding volunteers for a starvation study could have been a huge challenge (and would not be considered ethical today), but in the U.S. at the time there happened to be thousands of conscientious objectors (COs), who had been assigned public service in lieu of military duty. Among the forms of service they could sign up for was participating in medical experiments.

Keys got approval from the War Department to recruit COs as volunteers, and he and his team selected a group of young men they deemed models of psychological and physical fitness. By all accounts, these volunteers were remarkably well-adjusted people before they enrolled; as the experiment progressed... not so much. The researchers put the men on a six-month diet calculated to meet just over half their food needs.

The researchers referred to this as a "semi-starvation diet."

There was nothing "semi" about its effects.

On the diet these previously happy men became irritable, anxious, depressed, emotionally unpredictable, and unable to concentrate. They binged on their meager rations, hoarded food, and engaged in other odd food rituals. They became obsessed with food, dreaming and fantasizing about it constantly. Physically, they experienced dizziness, lethargy, weakness, hair loss, decreased tolerance for cold temperatures, and a dramatic reduction in sex drive.

Two volunteers were kicked out of the experiment because they broke the diet: one was caught stealing and eating raw rutabagas, the other eating *garbage scraps*. Both men suffered severe psychological distress, occasioning brief stays in the psychiatric ward of the university hospital. Neither had shown signs of mental illness before the diet; their psychological changes resulted from starvation.

I typically don't like to talk about calories because they're so tied up with diet culture, and I certainly won't use numbers here, but I will say this: the calorie count the Minnesota subjects were allowed during their hellish six-month experience equals that of a particularly *generous* diet today. Most diets promoted by women's magazines and diet-book authors contain far less. As one 2015 study aptly put it, "The level of energy intake recommended by many popular diets is comparable to that of the most undernourished global regions, where severe hunger interferes with individuals' ability to thrive and make meaningful contributions to society."[4]

Even if modern women have lower average energy needs than the young men in the Minnesota study (debatable—some women need a lot more food than those men, because everyone's body is different and individual energy requirements are hard to predict[5]), the low-calorie diets peddled to women fail to meet the needs of *their* bodies by a significant degree, putting them at risk of the same outcomes as the study subjects. So if you've ever felt you were losing your mind on a diet, the Minnesota Starvation Experiment shows you're not alone—and that food deprivation is the cause. It's not your fault that your mental health has suffered on diets; it's hard to feel happy and carefree when you're ready to gouge someone's eye out for a piece of bread.

Not only does diet culture thwart the physical need for nourishment, it prevents us from satisfying our basic psychological needs. According to a leading school of thought in psychology, there are three universal psychological needs: autonomy, competence, and relatedness.[6] When all three are met, we feel a sense of happiness and emotional well-being. When any of those needs are denied, however, we experience a decline in happiness and a greater likelihood of negative psychological outcomes such as depression and anxiety.

Diet culture sabotages our ability to meet these fundamental needs.

First, it dismisses our need for autonomy, making us feel we can't trust ourselves to make our own choices about food and movement. We have our own instincts about these things, and when we have the opportunity to tune back in to them they can lead us to the well-being we long for. Yet with diet culture constantly screaming in our ears, we're never allowed to get there. Think that sandwich looks good for lunch? Diet culture's like, *Sorry, that's got gluten and dairy in it, which will immediately kill you.* Feel like taking a nice walk and enjoying some sunshine? Diet culture's all, *Nope, not good enough—you need to get that heart rate up if you want to stop looking like such a beast.* How about a slice of cake at the office birthday party? [Smacks plate out of your hands] *It's a good thing you've got me around to save you from yourself.*

All the autonomy and agency we were born with when it comes to food—knowing when we were hungry and telling the world about it, eating what looked good and being excited to try new things, losing interest in food when we'd had enough, moving our bodies whenever we felt like it and resting when we needed to—got taken away as we were indoctrinated into diet culture. Instead of relying on our inner wisdom about what, when, and how much to eat and move, we've been conditioned to believe that some authority knows better—whether that's Dr. Oz or Grandpa Google, our moms or our holistic nutritionists. We've allowed the so-called "experts" to run our lives when it comes to food and movement, and as a society we're suffering for it. Millions of people see their need for autonomy thwarted multiple times a day—every time, that is, they think about what to eat and subject themselves to the Life Thief's rules and restrictions.

Second, diet culture undermines our sense of competence. It makes us think *we're* the failure when diets don't work, or when they inevitably lead to psychological distress and other nasty effects on our health. Diet culture's insidious rhetoric makes it seem like millions of people are having wild success on any given "program" or "protocol," and therefore if you're having trouble with it *you're* the problem. This tactic makes you blame yourself, which is great for diet culture's bottom line but terrible for your emotional well-being. Feeling like a failure can shake you at a deep psychological level, thwarting your need for competence and causing intense shame.

Even people who are wildly accomplished in other areas of their lives (think Oprah) can feel like such disappointments when it comes to food and their bodies that they sign over decades of their lives—and thousands upon thousands (or in Oprah's case, millions) of dollars—to diet culture. I've had far too many brilliant, hardworking, conscientious clients tell me, "I must be doing something wrong, because I'm still fat." Or, "I've cut out every food under the sun and I'm still having symptoms—I think my body is broken." As Oprah put it in 2009, all the success in the world "doesn't mean anything if you can't fit into your clothes. I am mad at myself. I am embarrassed."[7] This self-blame causes a tremendous amount of unnecessary pain, given that diet culture is the real failure here.

Third and finally, diet culture frustrates our need for relatedness, stigmatizing people whose bodies or eating habits fall outside the supposed ideal. Research has shown that public-health efforts to get people to "eat better" and lose weight have resulted in a society that's more divided, with more unequal treatment of people in larger bodies and those who don't engage in so-called "healthy" behaviors.[8] That's in addition to the stigma and exclusion people in larger bodies feel when they can't shop in mainstream clothing stores with their smaller-bodied friends, or fit comfortably in seats at theaters, restaurants, and airplanes. Indeed, so intense is the stigma heaped on people who don't meet diet culture's impossible standards that even people with what we in the anti-diet field refer to as *thin privilege* are conditioned to fear ostracism if they don't maintain their thinness or their Wellness Diet–approved food choices.

Granted, diet culture can create a sense of relatedness and

community with others pursuing the same "program" or "proto-col," which is why Weight Watchers meetings (er, WW "Wellness Workshops") and Paleo message boards can feel so welcoming to people on those diets—and why casual conversations these days tend to revolve around who's doing keto or cutting out glu-ten. When I first discovered dieting, it gave me a newfound sense of connection to others—particularly other women—that I desperately needed. That was a time in my life when I was feel-ing unmoored, having just returned from studying abroad and broken up with my long-term boyfriend, and panicking about my impending graduation and what I was going to do with my life. I craved a sense of belonging, and dieting seemed to give it to me. There is a sneaky sort of fake comfort that comes from being able to share cauliflower-rice recipes and pretend together that you enjoy them. But as many of us who've become disillu-sioned with diets know, the feeling of relatedness that comes from dieting is a false one, contingent as it is on staying on the diet or in the program. The faux bond hinges on continuing to do something that's harming you. When people realize diets don't work and leave groups like this, they may lose the relation-ships they formed there; at best, these relationships tend to become strained by the difference in values. For many of my cli-ents, hearing their keto or Beachbody pals talk incessantly about weight, food, and exercise is too much to bear when they're try-ing to heal their relationships with food and their bodies. Trips home to visit a dieting family are fraught with uncomfortable conversations and comparisons.

If you're dieting but your close friends and family are not, meanwhile, it can lead to a sense of superiority yet also a sense of isolation. Friendships suffer when one person suddenly spends all their time at the gym, or when they're too preoccupied with nutrition and health to be present in a conversation. And, as I've mentioned, getting locked into obsessive rules about food makes it hard to go out to eat with people anymore. For anyone who's had weight-loss surgery, going to restaurants can bring added layers of discomfort: being able to eat only a tiny amount of food at a time, having to watch other people eat things you wish you could try, and running to the bathroom when surgery complications such as dumping syndrome strike.

That's not even to mention how diet culture affects your romantic relationships. One Valentine's Day, Katie Dalebout and her boyfriend at the time drove an hour and a half in the snow to a raw-vegan restaurant—one of the only places in the area with more than a few menu options she would allow herself to eat. When they arrived, though, the restaurant was closed. It was too late to find another health-food restaurant that fit Dalebout's strict diet, and by this point she was really hungry. "We ended up going to some place where I got shredded lettuce with no cheese—one of those salads from, like, a sports bar that had nothing on it, because that was the only thing I would eat," she says. "He said to me once, 'You care more about food than you do about me,' and it was true. It was so true." Being caught up in diet culture can make food seem like the most important thing in your life—to the detriment of any human vying for that position.

Additionally, for everyone living in diet culture and especially for folks living in larger bodies, romantic relationships can be fraught with body-image concerns. Often people put their dating lives on hold until they lose weight, which means years of wasted time that could have been spent with someone they loved, instead of with a head full of diet rules. And when people finally dive into the dating pool, the waters can be rough. Weight-based trolling happens on dating websites because people can be just as awful there as anywhere else. I've heard horror stories from my friends and clients in larger bodies about some of the awful, bigoted things that have been said to them on dating sites and apps.

Even when you aren't actively being trolled by some garbage monster on Tinder, you can unconsciously do it to yourself. Internalized weight stigma can make you feel like you don't deserve to date or find love, compelling you to second-guess any interest from potential romantic partners. It can shut down your ability to be present and get to know someone on a human level. "Before I found body positivity, it would have been impossible for me to look at any of our encounters or dates in a way that wasn't, 'Is he looking at my stomach?' 'Is he noticing that I'm fat?'" says writer and body-positivity advocate Sophia Carter-Kahn of her long-term partner. Fortunately, because of her own work to embrace body acceptance, she was able to put those fears aside—and ask for reassurance from her partner when she needed it—to build a relationship unclouded by self-consciousness. Her experience is sadly a rare one, though; for too many people in diet culture, worries about their bodies act like a wedge in relationships.

This is especially true when it comes to sexuality, because feeling bad about your body can wreak havoc on your sex life. "Negative body image affects all domains of sexual functioning and satisfaction," says Melissa A. Fabello, an educator with a PhD in human sexuality studies. "We live in a fatphobic society where if we feel like we're fat, then we're less likely to feel good about our bodies—and that of course has a huge impact on how we engage in our sexual relationships." Fabello explains that women who feel bad about their bodies are less likely to undress in front of their partners, less likely to have sex with the lights on, and less adventurous and open in the bedroom, all of which can lower satisfaction overall. She points to a recent *Cosmopolitan* survey that found one-third of women are unable to have orgasms because they're too "in their head" or focused on how they look.

That was definitely my occasional experience when I was

caught up in diet culture. Other times it was, um, a little different: in the most restrictive depths of my disordered eating, I had a brief period when I fantasized about food during sex. That had never happened before I started dieting, and hasn't since I recovered. Food became a temporary fetish because I was so deprived of it. "I can't recall having come across that in my own research," Fabello said. "But it doesn't surprise me that you would have that experience."

"Emotional Eating" and Diet Culture

When diet culture undermines your happiness in all these ways, it's natural to look for solace. Many people in this situation turn to food for comfort, which diet culture labels as "emotional eating." Here's the really insidious part: while diet culture blames this behavior for ruining your diet or "plan" and shames you for engaging in it, *dieting and restrictive eating itself* is the force driving most people toward comfort food. So-called emotional eating is in fact a response to the deprivation caused by dieting.

Under normal circumstances (*not* dieting), people respond to difficult emotions by losing their appetite. For nondieters, a lack of interest in food is a common symptom of grief, depression, and anxiety, among other negative emotions. This makes sense from a biological standpoint: in the short term, our ability to respond to something bad happening is more important for our survival than eating is. In those situations, we're programmed to stop thinking about food and start dealing with the matter at hand. Eventually, once we've recovered from the initial emotional blow (or, in our ancestors' case, eluded that angry lion), we start thinking about food again.

With chronic dieters, though, something contrary happens: negative emotions provoke an *increased* appetite and desire to eat.[9] Dieters develop the response opposite to what we see in intuitive eaters. Psychologists believe this is because for dieters, eating is under conscious cognitive control (as opposed to intuitive eaters, who take their eating cues from their bodies and exert no cognitive effort to control their intake), and negative emotions disrupt and deplete that cognitive control. Once the inhibition is gone, the appetite that was being suppressed emerges in a big way, like Roger Rabbit bursting through a brick wall. Negative emotions inadvertently break down the barriers that were holding dieters back from their true desire to eat.

Not only that, but restrained eating can *cause* an increase in negative emotions. The Minnesota Starvation Experiment participants are a prime example of how the physical deprivation created by dieting increases people's risk of mental-health challenges. More recent research has confirmed that dieters—even those who wouldn't necessarily identify as such, but simply "watch what they eat"—are more likely than intuitive eaters to suffer from depression, low self-esteem, disordered eating, and overall psychological distress.[10]

As I've seen both in my clinical practice and in my own life, what people label as emotional eating is often just a completely understandable response to deprivation. The behavior disappears—or at least is dramatically reduced—when they break free from diet culture's rules and restrictions. Many (and I would guess even most) people who identify as emotional eaters don't need to learn how to cope with their feelings without using food; they just need to learn how to cope with their eating without using diets.

In fact, decades of psychological research on emotional eating has shown that it may not be a scientifically sound concept; in experimental settings, self-identified emotional eaters don't eat any more in the presence of emotional stimuli than anyone else.[11] Instead, people who identify as emotional eaters seem to be simply more *worried* about their eating behavior, feel they lack control over it, and follow external rules about "healthy eating." There's also evidence that people who see themselves as emotional eaters have a greater tendency to attribute any perceived overeating to emotions.

Why do so many people worry about so-called emotional eating? That would be because of diet culture, which has a deep investment in making you feel like your eating is driven by "mere emotions" instead of by legitimate needs that diets will never meet. Diet culture has a major stake in making you feel like a failure instead of knowing the truth: that *diets themselves* are the failure. The concept of emotional eating emerged in the 1960s, and Weight Watchers and other diet companies did a deft job of disseminating it. It was an ingenious way to pass the buck, deflecting attention from the fact that dieting made people feel unhinged around food.

If we can pull back from diet culture and stop letting it control us, we'll see that there's no reason to demonize the practice of eating to soothe emotions—*and* that when we truly heal from dieting and deprivation, we likely won't "eat our feelings" as much anymore.

For many people who identify as emotional eaters, finding additional ways to cope with difficult emotions is important, too. Some folks have labeled themselves as emotional eaters for so long that they don't have many other tools in their coping toolboxes; if that describes you, adding more of these tools can help address the vast array of feelings and situations that might come up over the years. That's not to say you must stop turning to food for comfort—not at all; it's simply a matter of *adding* more coping skills so you feel better equipped to deal with life.

Diet culture's MO is to say, "Take a bath *instead* of eating." But I'm saying, "How about you call a friend after you finish that ice cream—and PS, who takes baths anymore?"* With enough practice at intuitive eating (which we'll discuss shortly), the desire to eat in response to emotions will decline on its own. In the meantime, there's absolutely nothing wrong with eating if that's what you feel like doing when you're bummed out—and if you're recovering from chronic dieting, you probably will.

Bottom line? If you identify as an emotional eater, it's not your fault; it's the fault of diet culture. It's perfectly OK to eat for emotional reasons rather than strictly biological ones. Plus how can you really distinguish between the two? Dieting and restricting foods creates such a chronic sense of deprivation that there's almost always some hunger going on, some physical need not being met. Sometimes that deprivation is what's driving the emotions: chronic food deprivation will make *anyone* cranky, sad, and anxious. So instead of trying to substitute other coping mechanisms for eating every time you find yourself soothing a feeling with food, try instead to stop demonizing emotional eating—and stop following diet culture's rules. You may still comfort yourself with food sometimes, and that's a completely normal part of a peaceful relationship with food.

In the words of health coach Isabel Foxen Duke: "I don't really give a shit that sometimes I want to eat a brownie when I'm sad." Even the most intuitive eater occasionally eats in an "emotional" way—and there's nothing wrong with that.

---

* Kidding! I'm sure plenty of people still take baths, and I've been known to do it myself from time to time (when I'm at a hotel, for instance, and the tub is squeaky clean). But so many old-school anti-emotional-eating gurus recommend taking a bath instead of eating that it's become a running joke among some of my colleagues and clients. Baths are nice and all, but there are so many other ways to comfort yourself that don't require scrubbing out a dingy old tub.

*　　*　　*

It's clear that diet culture has robbed millions of us of our happiness—not to mention our time, our money, and our well-being—in all kinds of subtle and not-so-subtle ways. Life outside diet culture is rich and full, with more possibilities than you could ever imagine when you're in that narrow place of thinking about food and your body 24/7. This brave new world beyond dieting is what we'll turn to next.

PART II

Life Beyond Diet Culture

CHAPTER 7

Enough Is Enough

When you start to realize everything that diet culture has taken from you, and all the ways it's still sneaking around in the corners of your mind, it's common to be pissed. You've been cheated with false promises of permanent weight loss and perfect health, and it's understandable to feel enraged about that. You were doing exactly what you were told to do, and it didn't work—through no fault of your own, but because the instructions you got were lies.

Getting angry at diet culture is an important part of the healing process—a powerful antidote to the inward-directed anger that the Life Thief creates to distract you from its crimes. Because make no mistake: beating yourself up for "failing" to lose weight and keep it off—or for not being able to stick to a diet of exclusively "whole," "unprocessed" foods—distracts you from what should be the real object of our collective anger, which is diet culture itself. Listening to diet culture's rhetoric, it's easy to think *I'm bad, I'm terrible, I have this problem with food, it's all my fault.* But that overlooks all the research (and your lived experience) showing that playing by diet culture's rules doesn't work in the long run.

By training us to blame ourselves when diets don't work, the Life Thief keeps us from turning our rage and blame on *it.* That's why there's something incredibly powerful and transformative about putting your foot down and saying, "Enough is enough"—reclaiming that anger and directing it toward diet culture, where it belongs, instead of staying in a cycle of self-loathing that keeps you spending more and more of your precious time, money, and energy on diet culture's bullshit products and programs. Recognizing and naming the Life Thief for what it is—and feeling the righteous anger that comes with that naming—ultimately empowers you to distance yourself from diet culture and reclaim your life.

Anger gets a bad rap in our society, though—particularly for women and femmes, who've been conditioned to suppress our anger and let it out only in small, passive-aggressive ways. Terms such as *hysterical, shrill, nagging, bitchy,* and *drama queen* get lobbed at lady-folks who dare to express anger about the injustices we face in the world—sexist comments while we're walking down the street, the pay gap, limited reproductive rights, political disenfranchisement for women and femmes of color. We have endless reasons to be enraged, yet we're told over and over again that our ire is unacceptable. And so we learn to push the anger down, to soften the edges we show to the world, to turn the sharpest points in on ourselves. As feminist writer Laurie Penny puts it, "The patriarchy is so scared of women's anger that eventually we learn to fear it, too. We walk around as if we were bombs about to go off, worried about admitting how livid we really are, even to ourselves."[1]

Psychotherapist Carmen Cool says this is a common fear whenever we feel anger, or any other emotion that we know runs deep: when we allow ourselves to tap into our rage about one thing, it can put us in touch with a whole network of other things we're pissed off about. When it comes to your anger about diet culture, then, it's understandable that you might feel scared to let it out, for fear of being engulfed. But you don't have to feel or express it all at once. You can take your time. "One of my teachers used to talk about the idea of 'touch and go,'" Cool says. "We can touch into a feeling and then we can move back out of it—we don't have to go farther than we feel safe to." You can process it little by little, and you can enlist the support of people in your life to help—people who can, as Cool puts it, "reflect us back to ourselves."

Inevitably someone will suggest you shouldn't let all this diet-culture stuff "get to you"—that you should turn the other cheek, that anger is no way to respond to injustice, that you should "rise above" your anger. Quite a few of my clients have a naysaying voice like this in their lives, and it can be incredibly confusing. Whereas this kind of advice usually comes from a well-intentioned place, its effect is to dismiss and invalidate your feelings. But I can assure you that the anger you feel is valid—and justified. You have every right to be pissed off. "Your anger is necessary," Cool says.

It's also normal to be sad when you realize everything diet culture stole from you. Indeed, many people go through a mourning process when they wake up to that. "I was mad as hell for a while, and I was really sad, and I was depressed for a period of time," says Kathleen Bishop, a clinical social worker who went through her own recovery from diet culture after being stuck in it for about forty years. "I had all the stages of grief, not in any particular order, going back and forth," she says. In fact, sadness and anger aren't as distinct as our society makes them out to be. They're two sides of the same coin; it's just that we're socialized in our society to show only one side. People assigned female at birth (AFAB) are raised to show only sadness, whereas people assigned male at birth (AMAB) are raised to show only anger. Women and AFAB folks are conditioned to privilege sadness over anger—to deny our pissed-off feelings and, if we're going to allow ourselves the free expression of any emotions at all, to give voice only to our pain, which is much more culturally accepted for feminine folks than anger.

As Leslie Jamison wrote in a 2018 article for the *New York Times*, "It has always been easier to shunt female sadness and female anger into the 'watertight compartments' of opposing archetypes, rather than acknowledging the ways they run together in the cargo hold of every female psyche."[2] Dealing with hardship or oppression can make us feel enraged and despondent— either at the same time or, as Bishop describes, in cyclical succession. When it comes to diet culture, we might feel angry at having done exactly what we thought we were supposed to do but having ended up with results opposite those we were promised, while also grieving for our younger self who missed out on so many beautiful moments in life because of diet culture. We might simultaneously feel the pain of having been betrayed and rage toward the betrayer. As Jamison writes, "No woman's anger is an island."

Bishop still gets angry sometimes when she imagines what her life might have been if she'd never had to struggle with food and body-image issues. Now, though, she has an outlet for her anger: advocacy and activism.

Anger as Power

> Every woman has a well-stocked arsenal of anger potentially useful against those oppressions, personal and institutional, which brought that anger into being. Focused with precision it can become a powerful source of energy serving progress and change.
>
> — AUDRE LORDE

Though long-suppressed emotions can feel overwhelming when we first begin acknowledging them, our anger toward diet culture (or toward anything, really) isn't a flood that will inevitably drown us; instead, it's a wave that we can learn to surf and to channel. The key is to not fight against the anger and get stuck in a vortex of self-loathing, but instead to let the rage move through us without judging it. When you find yourself atop a wave of anger, just stay present and ride it to the shore. To help you do that, Cool recommends asking yourself questions such as *What is the healing impulse inside my anger?* or *What is my anger telling me about what needs to be different?* or *What does my anger want to communicate?* Listen to what your anger is telling you and it will let you know how to proceed in the most self-caring way possible.

Cool remembers how that fiery compassion got ignited for her in her own early stages of recovery: "I started thinking about the way my dreams had been slipping away from me, and then I started thinking about how that's true for so many people, and I started thinking about all the things that we could be doing in the world if we had our energy back, if we had our time back from spending it on some project of trying to be a body we think we're supposed to be—that if we reoriented all of that energy back into the world, so much more would be possible," she says. "And when I really started thinking about that, I just started getting really pissed off at all of the forces that told me I wasn't OK just as I was. I felt like I wanted to start fighting back in some way. I wanted to start reclaiming my right to be in my body just as it was. Not that that was an instant switch, but my desire to reclaim that was strong."

She has brought that fierceness into her therapy practice as well. Unlike psychotherapists in the traditional Freudian model, which requires the therapist to maintain a blank-slate detachment, Cool (despite her name) is a proponent of showing her emotions—anger included—in a therapeutic setting. "Anger and outrage has a place," she says, "and sometimes that can be the most skillful thing and the most useful thing and frankly the most loving thing I can offer. Anger is such an immediate source of information and holds so much wisdom. It lets us know if a boundary is being crossed, it alerts us when something is going on that is not good for us or someone else, or it lets us know that something needs to stop. If our anger is in response to something we need to say no to, it calls forward the part of us that is our own ally. We may not always know what to do next, but feeling the *no* puts us in contact with our sense of who we are and what we need."

Eventually your anger will pass, just like every emotion—and then it will resurface again, also like every emotion. That ebb and flow will continue for your whole life, and that's normal. With practice, we can learn to use the power of our anger to propel us forward in the fight for justice.

That's exactly what happened for Joy Cox, a communications researcher who studies social movements and political action. In 2013, when she was in the early stages of a PhD program, Cox saw a report on the evening news that the American Medical Association had officially classified "obesity" as a disease. "I remember being so upset and so angry, because I've lived in this fat body my whole life, and I've never considered myself [diseased]," she says. Outraged, she called her sister, hoping to vent her anger and get some support. Unfortunately, her sister "didn't get it," Cox says.

So she sat with her rage, mulling what to do with it. Cox recognized this was something she felt passionate about on both a personal and an intellectual level. She got curious about how the discourse on body size had come to this point, and she realized it was something she could study for her PhD thesis. "In that moment, I changed my research trajectory," Cox says. She went on to write a dissertation about the discourse around fatness within and outside the fat-acceptance movement, deepening the wealth of academic literature in this area. And she became active in the movement herself, joining organizations promoting size acceptance and starting her own podcast where she speaks out about fat liberation. Cox channeled her anger into action.

The same is true for Rachel Roberts, an actor and playwright based in Sydney, Australia, and a participant in my intuitive eating online course. As she was working toward making peace with food and her body, Roberts found herself getting angrier and angrier at the culture that had triggered her disordered eating. So she decided to direct that anger into her art, and wrote a one-woman show about it called *Everything You Ever Wanted*. The piece explored the truth about weight science and weight stigma as well as her own troubled history with food, with some fun audience interaction peppered in. It was very well received; a review in the Sydney-based performing-arts magazine *Audrey Journal* called the show "compassionate and pragmatic, with a satisfyingly sharp bite."

That bite, Roberts says, came directly from her own feelings. "My anger — and need for solidarity, and fear, and hurt — fueled my show, which I'm so proud of," she says. That anger fuels her in everyday life, too: "My anger helps me stand up to diet culture. When a comment scares and upsets me, my anger is the palm on my back pushing me to say something — even if it's not perfect, even if I get upset when speaking."

Psychologist Rachel Millner likewise experienced anger as a palm on her back, guiding her toward a career helping others recover. As she recounted in Chapter 5, she struggled with anorexia in her twenties, but no one diagnosed it until she became emaciated — at which point she'd been suffering for years. Even at the time, that pissed her off. "I knew I wanted to be a psychologist from the time I was pretty young, and I was angry about the ways that I was harmed — I had many medical providers and mental-health providers who were stigmatizing and said things about my body that were not OK," she says. "So as I recovered, I really wanted to be able to offer a different kind of care." She has gone on to build her career around helping people — particularly adolescents — recover from eating disorders, weight stigma, and diet culture, whatever their size. The clients she now advocates for are in much the same position Millner was in when she went through her recovery; thanks to her, however, they're hearing a far different message than the one she got in treatment. "For people who are living in larger bodies and are struggling with anorexia, or really with any eating disorder, what they are going through is important and it matters," she says. "They deserve empathy and help and care and support the same way somebody in a smaller body does. They deserve that and are entitled to it."

I very much identify with Millner's anger about being overlooked and misdiagnosed by health-care providers. When I was hopping from doctor to doctor in my early twenties, trying to figure out why my period had been missing for months, not a single physician, nurse, or therapist recognized that restrictive eating and overexercise were causing my hormonal abnormalities. Someone definitely should've picked up on that, and the fact that they didn't is 100 percent due to diet culture and the weight stigma it creates. Because my BMI was still in the so-called "normal" range, my doctors never suspected that dieting and disordered-eating behaviors could be the root of my problems. (The vast majority of people with eating issues don't resemble the stereotypical picture of an eating disorder; in fact, many people who match diet culture's supposed picture of "health" are locked in a painful struggle with food and their bodies.)

When I started to understand these facts and recognize that the care I'd received was woefully inadequate, it filled me with rage—and spurred me to action. My anger at the injustice that I and so many others had faced motivated me to focus my journalism and nutrition work on disordered eating and recovery. It helped me overcome my introverted tendencies enough to start sharing my story publicly. It gave me a reason to keep fighting and pushing for change, even though it would've been so much easier (not to mention more lucrative) to roll over and sell weight-loss regimens as most dietitians do, or to keep writing stories about "seven foods to avoid" as most health and nutrition journalists do. Anger is what motivated me to learn about and understand diet culture. If it weren't for my anger, you wouldn't be holding this book in your hands right now.

In other words: anger helps us get shit *done*.

Short of a career shift or public statement, you can express your anger toward diet culture in plenty of small, private ways. "I've found that in this journey of making peace with food, actually feeling my feelings has been one of the most difficult and crucial steps," says Molly, one of my course participants. "I will often ask myself, *What am I feeling right now?* And a lot of the time I will feel angry when it comes to negative-body-image days and guilt/shame associated with food." Just naming that anger and giving yourself permission to feel it can help you release it, rather than keeping it directed inward where it does harm. "It feels really good that I no longer need to place that anger upon myself, but that I can throw all of it at the very deserving diet culture that surrounds us," Molly says. "I don't usually swear, but saying 'FUCK YOU, DIET CULTURE!' has seriously been one of the most helpful phrases when trying to feel my feelings and cultivate my anti-diet passion."

That fuck-you energy is essential for recovering from diet culture and reclaiming our relationships with food. "Someone asked me recently what the single most important factor was for me in recovering from my eating disorder," says psychotherapist Cool, who struggled with diet-culture thinking and disordered eating throughout her childhood and into college. "While I wanted to say that it was compassion, or love, the truth is that it was outrage. The anger that surfaces can get us looking for another alternative."

Getting pissed off at the way the Life Thief has led you astray can help clarify what you really want out of life. It can make you commit to finding a different path. As Jenny, another one of my course participants, confides: "When confronted with weight stigma, I used to feel this crushing and intense 'not-enoughness' and would try to shrink myself. I wanted nothing more than to disappear and felt apologetic for my size. However, since educating myself on what intuitive eating really is and how weight stigma has robbed not only me but my mother, my brother, my best friend, and *so many* other people of happiness, I get angry. I don't want to retreat. I want to enlighten society and highlight how detrimental it is to stigmatize those in larger bodies."

Getting angry about diet culture and the weight stigma it creates can also help sustain your recovery long-term. Take therapist Amy Pershing, for example. Even though she's decades into recovery, fully accepts her body, and helps people recover from diet culture *for a living*, the occasional self-stigmatizing thought still flashes through her brain: *I shouldn't wear this because I don't look thin in it,* for example. "I still have those thoughts crop up because that wiring is so old and so deep," Pershing says. "But now when it triggers, instead of feeling shame, what I feel is anger. It makes me mad [that I went through it] and it makes me mad for my clients. It makes me mad when I see people on Facebook posting how much weight they've lost on their latest diet since the New Year or whatever. It just makes me sad and it makes me angry and that's OK—I'm OK with that reaction."

I have a similar response whenever those thoughts cross my own mind. Whereas I, too, am a professional anti-diet activist many years into recovery, body-negative thoughts still pop up occasionally for me as well. Unlike during my disordered-eating days, though, now I notice when those thoughts are happening (instead of being unconsciously pulled along by them) and can identify their source: diet culture. Then I think about what a fucking tragedy it is that *all* of us got brainwashed with these kinds of harmful thoughts at a young age, and pretty quickly I'm able to move past the self-judgment and reconnect with my sense of common humanity and my commitment to taking down diet culture. Sometimes I put my hand on whatever body part I'm currently feeling less-than-awesome about and mentally say, *I love you*. Sometimes I literally say out loud into the mirror, "Fuck diet culture. You're amazing."

In that sense, feeling and acknowledging my anger toward the Life Thief helps me become more compassionate toward myself and others. Rage transforms into fierce love.

The Importance of Self-Compassion

Speaking of being compassionate toward yourself, that's an essential part of healing from diet culture. Anger toward the Life Thief is healing; anger toward yourself is not. You don't need to beat yourself up for having fallen into its traps, because we live in diet culture and the traps are *everywhere* (and millions of us have fallen into them, too). If you've engaged in disordered eating and dieting as a response to all the oppressive forces telling you to do exactly that, you're only human. And if you want to lose weight in this culture, you're certainly not alone — it's what we've all been told to want for our whole lives.

In fact, berating yourself for getting conned by the Life Thief only adds to the problem. Research shows that shame is a terrible motivator for recovering from disordered-eating and body-image issues — you can't rebuke yourself into loving your body or shame yourself into a peaceful relationship with food.[3] As I learned the hard way, punishing yourself — for, say, bingeing on chips at your family picnic because you'd been trying to avoid carbs all week — only makes that pattern more likely to repeat itself. A much better approach is self-compassion, which means acknowledging your feelings (including anger) without judgment, being kind and caring toward yourself even when you want to change some aspect of your behavior, and recognizing that *all* human beings struggle and feel inadequate sometimes.[4]

Self-compassion interventions have been shown to improve

body satisfaction, and higher levels of self-compassion are associated with lower levels of disordered-eating behavior.[5] So when you're working to escape from diet culture, it behooves you to be nice to yourself, and to direct your anger where it really belongs. Whenever diet-culture thoughts pop into your mind, remember it's not your fault—it's the Life Thief's fault, and it's going to take time, practice, and support to escape its grip. Give yourself the space you need, and don't expect to be free from diet culture overnight.

One skill to help you break free is setting boundaries, and it definitely takes practice to master.

Setting Boundaries

Real talk: I didn't even know what boundaries *were* for the first twenty-eight years or so of my life. I just had this low-level rage simmering all the time, because I was getting my boundaries violated left and right without even realizing it. Many AFAB people in our society are in the same position—but it turns out that boundaries are a key concept for psychological functioning. At the most basic level, boundaries are a way of drawing a line between ourselves and others. When it comes to diet culture, boundaries are a way of saying *Enough!* to the Life Thief's bullshit (or *anybody's* bullshit, really). They come from a place of self-compassion—a recognition that we truly deserve to listen to and honor our own needs and desires, as does every other human being on this planet. As Renée, a participant in my online course, aptly puts it, "Boundaries are a *NO* that comes from healthy, grounded anger (as opposed to rage, which is more like an out-of-control combination of fear and anger)." Setting boundaries means communicating our needs to other people, speaking out when those needs aren't met, and taking care of ourselves. Too often, AFAB folks allow people to do and say things that hurt us, because we've been socialized to "be nice" and "go with the flow." But when we set boundaries, we're able to make it clear what kind of rhetoric and behavior we will and won't accept from other people.

Setting boundaries might mean putting a moratorium on diet talk with your mother, or asking your doctor to stop recommending weight loss (and switching doctors if they won't). It can mean unfollowing friends on social media who constantly post about their keto diets and Whole30s, or unsubscribing from the email list of every diet program and "wellness expert" you've worked with over the years. Setting boundaries can also mean standing up against weight stigma just like you'd stand up against racism and sexism, or telling your best friend you won't be joining them for the dance class with the fatphobic teacher anymore. In order to deal with the inevitable diet culture that pops up in various aspects of life, from work meetings to playdates, you need to learn to say no in a million different ways.

Boundary setting is a form of self-care, but diet culture systematically negates our need for self-care and replaces it with self-control. Diet culture teaches us we don't deserve to care for ourselves or have our needs met. It tells us that the food our bodies need and want is "too much," "unhealthy," or just plain "bad." It tells us that it's our fault if we're getting disrespected for the size or shape of our bodies—and that if we're currently getting the respect we *all* truly deserve, it could disappear if we gain weight. It tells us we don't deserve fun, rest, or comfort unless and until we fit into an impossible ideal of what bodies "should" look like. Diet culture disconnects us from our own needs and shames us for having them.

No wonder so many of us have a hard time asking for and getting what we need. No wonder we have a hard time setting boundaries in the first place.

So it's important to know that setting boundaries feels uncomfortable, awkward, and scary at first. When we've been socialized to think we don't deserve to stand up for ourselves or have our needs met, it takes a lot of time, practice, and support to get used to drawing those lines with people. "When you don't have self-esteem, setting boundaries is the scariest thing ever," says Victoria Welsby, now a body-positive activist and life coach who endured a tremendous amount of trauma around food and weight early in her life and suffered from extremely low self-confidence as a result. "I remember the first time trying out setting boundaries and it being absolutely fucking terrifying, and presuming that people's responses would be like, 'How dare you ask for this, you bastard!'" But in fact, most of the time it wasn't like that at all. "People's reactions were like, 'Yeah, sure,'" Welsby says.

Of course, occasionally people don't take it quite so well when you set boundaries. "Sometimes people don't react positively, and then [you] realiz[e] that's them; it's nothing to do with me," Welsby says. Setting boundaries isn't unkind—if anything, it's a hell of a lot kinder to *yourself* than the alternative—but when the people in your life have been accustomed to your boundary-less ways, they might not be on board with the change right away. That doesn't mean you're wrong to set boundaries; it just means that your friends and family are going to need to get used to the new you. When it comes to diet culture, most of us spent years of our lives where we were happy to dish about our latest weight-loss plan or commiserate over the foods we were cutting out. Once you start thinking differently, it takes a while for the people in your life to get the memo and start adjusting how they talk to you—which might mean omitting discussions of body and weight altogether, at least for a while. The more steeped in diet culture these people are, the harder it'll be for them to honor your new boundaries, and they might be upset that they're losing their old dieting buddy. But that's not your fault, and it doesn't mean you should stop setting boundaries. Even though it may hurt to have to change the things you talk about and the ways you engage with the people in your life, the truly meaningful relationships will withstand those growing pains.

Likewise bear in mind that setting a boundary is only half the battle. The other half is *enforcing* the boundary, and that can take some repetition. Even when people really love you and want to do right by you, their fatphobic beliefs may be so deeply ingrained—and their diet talk so reflexive—that you need to constantly remind them of the boundary you set and explain how they've violated it. This doesn't mean they don't care about you, or that your boundary isn't valid (because it absolutely is); it simply means they're dealing with a lot of internalized diet-culture stuff themselves, and that's going to take some time.

Setting boundaries also means picking your battles—knowing when you feel up for engaging in a discussion about diet culture, and knowing when you need to take a break and excuse yourself from the conversation. "There's a time for me to engage, and the way that I engage is my work," says Dana Falsetti, a body-confidence activist and yoga teacher. "And there's a time for me to set a boundary and say, 'I see where you are on your path, and this is not where I am on my path, and I'm going to just keep going on mine.'" In other words, there's no need to educate people about the perils of diet culture in every single situation you're in. Instead, you can choose to change the subject, leave the room, or do anything else that would help you in that moment.

Some people just aren't ready to hear the anti-diet message. Fighting to educate those folks is an uphill battle that invariably ends up hurting you more than it helps them. I speak from experience: These days I have a liberal delete-and-block policy on my social-media pages for anyone who comes at me in a way that says they just want to fight and aren't truly interested in learning about the anti-diet approach. If someone exhibits genuine curiosity, I'm happy to engage as time allows; if they're defending diet culture and upholding bigoted beliefs about body size, though, I'm *not* here for it. In my personal life, sometimes I'll speak up when people espouse diet-culture beliefs; at other times I'll choose not to for my own self-care. At a party with extended family I might voice my philosophy when someone starts talking about their latest diet, or I might opt to change the subject or leave the room. If I'm getting my oil changed and I overhear the cashier talking to one of the mechanics about intermittent fasting, I'll probably bite my tongue—unless I'm feeling especially salty that day, in which case I may get involved. If someone passes judgment on my body, however, I feel obliged to speak up.

This last one cuts both ways: just as you wouldn't want someone commenting on your weight, don't comment on theirs. Compliments, counterintuitively, can be especially harmful. When we celebrate weight loss, we actually harm the person we're praising, as well as anyone else within earshot. I know that may sound a bit harsh, but the reality is that applauding weight loss for anyone reinforces weight stigma for everyone. It tells the person you're complimenting that their body was "bad" or "wrong" before, and that it's worthy of acclaim only now that it's smaller. And it tells anyone listening the same thing.

Not only that, but intentional weight loss tends to royally screw up people's relationships with food. As we've discussed throughout this book, it takes them further away from the health they're probably seeking. Many people who've lost weight intentionally have done it via disordered behaviors such as restriction, compulsive exercise, and deprivation. Even if they're approaching their weight-loss efforts in a seemingly "flexible" way right now, research shows they're likely to slip into more rigid styles of eating down the line.[6]

Praising people for weight loss, then, often means applauding them for disordered behaviors and a damaging relationship with food. That's not to say weight loss is always the product of disordered behaviors; it can also stem from health issues, grief, food insecurity, or any number of other factors. The point is that we really never know what someone has done—or what has happened to them—to make them lose weight. So when we compliment weight loss, we risk lauding something that's actually a terrible experience in someone's life.

Think of it as another crucial boundary to set: when we stop applauding weight loss, we stop passing judgment on other people's bodies. There are so many more interesting things to talk about. I know it can be incredibly hard to withhold a compliment when someone is asking for validation and praise, but there are ways to reassure them without cosigning their dieting behavior. If it's someone you're really close with, you can say something like, "You know I love you no matter *what* size your body is." That helps remind them they're so much more than their body, and that you DGAF about their "weight-loss journey"—in a kind way. If it's someone you're not so close with, try making the same point in a slightly less effusive way. You can also redirect the conversation toward a more pleasant subject, or politely excuse yourself.

Setting boundaries isn't just for the early stages of your anti-diet journey; for most of us, including professionals in this field, it's a lifelong commitment. "There are magazines I don't buy," says fellow anti-diet dietitian Marci Evans. "There are messages I don't read. There are blogs I would never go on to. I maintain my own kind of bubble—as much as I can manage it—of what allows me to feel good, what supports my overall health and well-being. I'm just as selective as I encourage my clients to be."

Ultimately, setting boundaries helps you channel your anger toward diet culture in a direction where it can do some good—for yourself and for others. As a participant in my online course named Devinia writes: "The diet industry knowingly traps us in a vicious cycle. It made me believe for many years that being black and larger-bodied was wrong. Getting angry at diet culture has allowed me to fight back. I've got a voice and can stand up to the diet industry. I can say no to fad diets and so-called wellness gurus telling me I'm not good enough. It's given me confidence I never thought I would have to appreciate and respect my body. I've learned to use self-care to look after myself rather than hatred. Getting angry at diet culture has allowed me to appreciate who I truly am."

CHAPTER 8

Reclaim Your Right to Eat Intuitively

Intuitive eating is the body's default mode. It's the way we were *born* to eat. It's our birthright—regardless of body size, race, ethnicity, gender identity, or nationality. Except in some rare congenital conditions that can alter babies' appetites, we all basically had the whole hunger thing on lock from the time we left the womb. We made *noise* when we were hungry to let people know we needed food, and we didn't feel the tiniest bit of shame about it. We demanded to have our needs met. We knew those needs were valid and didn't second-guess them; we never asked ourselves whether or not we were "really" hungry. We owned our hunger. No one had to teach us how to do that. It was programmed into our brains—the same way that baby sea turtles are programmed to skitter into the ocean right after they hatch on the beach. In fact, the drive to eat comes from our "reptilian brain"—the oldest part of the human brain in terms of evolutionary history, and the one we share with animals including reptiles.[1] Our reptilian brains take care of our survival needs through powerful instincts. Like all animals, we humans instinctually know how to honor our hunger.

As babies and toddlers we also took pleasure in food, enjoying the flavors in our formula or breast milk, and eventually solid foods. We relished the foods we liked and spoke up when we wanted more of them—again without feeling any self-judgment. We didn't have much use for foods we didn't like, turning our heads away and pursing our lips until (hopefully) our caregivers tried giving us something we did enjoy, or realized we were done. Once we were full and satisfied, we lost interest in food and turned our attention to other things—such as playing, moving our bodies when we felt like it, and resting when we needed to—until eventually our instinct to eat kicked in again, and the cycle started all over.

Watching my nephew as a toddler was a beautiful reminder of this natural process. Like pretty much every two-to-three-year-old I've met, he was a huge fan of ice cream, candy, and other sweet snacks, and he gleefully devoured them whenever he had the opportunity. Once he'd had his fill, though, you couldn't interest him in another bite. He'd turn his head away and grimace if you tried to "airplane" another spoonful toward him. At meals, as soon as he was satisfied, he'd pop up from his chair, ready to play. He'd go around to each adult at the table, tugging their arm to try to make them join him. "You all done," he'd say declaratively, with a grin—knowing that he was being silly because clearly we were *not* all done.

Early in life, we were intuitive eaters—and we can be again. We have the capacity to get back to a place where our relationships with food are as simple as they were when we were babies— where hunger and pleasure are nothing to be ashamed of, and where fullness is a signal that we can take our minds off food for a while, secure in the knowledge that it will be available again when we want it.

Of course, many factors can get in the way of that security, that simplicity—things that mess with our default mode. Diet culture is of course a big one, but circumstances such as poverty and medical trauma around food can also disrupt our intuitive connection with our bodies' innate wisdom about eating. Any situation that causes deprivation can shake our sense of safety and take us out of our default mode. Deprivation is the very real sense that food *won't* be available again when we want it—that we don't have enough. Deprivation makes hunger, pleasure, and fullness stop feeling safe and easy. Deprivation makes our relationships with food become complicated and tortured.

Diet culture creates a sense of deprivation in many ways, both subtle and less so. It tells us that our hunger is "wrong," that we shouldn't own it or (God forbid) make noise about it. It tells us that weight gain and larger bodies are "bad," and that weight loss and smaller bodies are "good." (Never mind that before about 150 years ago, Western culture and other societies around the world were saying *the exact opposite*.) Diet culture tells us that satisfaction and pleasure will destroy our health and lead to those "bad" things, too. It also demonizes fullness, branding it a sign that we've eaten "too much." Diet culture convinces us that honoring our hunger, seeking satisfaction, and feeling full will send us down the road to perdition. It tells us our instincts— the innate signals encoded into our reptilian brains—are bad and wrong. It makes us lose trust in ourselves.

And so we stop honoring our hunger. We stop meeting our needs for satisfaction and pleasure. We stop feeling confident in the knowledge that we'll be able to eat enough, and eat things we enjoy, the next time we're hungry. And so fullness stops feeling safe, too. Fullness stops being a signal that we can take our minds off food and turn our attention to other matters. It starts being something that we fear, something that we question and condemn. The Life Thief makes us feel out of control and lost around food—like we don't know which way is up. Remember the Restriction Pendulum from Chapter 3? This is one of the key ways diet culture robs us of the peaceful relationship with food that is our birthright. Through the deprivation that diet culture creates, we lose our connection to our inner wisdom and start to feel we can't be trusted around food—because every time we come within a few feet of a plate of cookies or a bag of chips, we end up polishing off the whole thing. Or, on the rare chance that we don't, we still think and obsess about food constantly. It haunts our dreams (and sometimes even our sex lives, as it did mine).

The good news is, now that we know how diet culture led us astray, we don't have to buy into it anymore. You *can* return to the peaceful, easy relationship with food that you deserve to have. It will take some work to unlearn all of diet culture's harmful rules. But with practice and support, you have the capacity and the *right* to break free from the Life Thief and reclaim your innate appetite.

Intuitive Eating and the Importance of Enough

The first key to reconnecting with your body's innate wisdom about food and movement is kicking diet culture to the curb. That means recognizing how it robs you of your precious time on this planet. It also means noticing all the subtle, sneaky ways diet culture shows up in your mind, and refusing to live by the Life Thief's rules any longer. It means allowing yourself to feel pissed off and sad about the life diet culture stole from you, and galvanized to fight back. Rejecting diet culture and getting rid of the beliefs you internalized from it is the hardest and most essential step in repairing your relationship with food. If you've found yourself agreeing with the case I've laid out so far, you're well on your way to healing from the diet mentality.

The second key to getting back to the default mode of intuitive eating is to help your body trust that you won't be depriving it anymore. Having *enough* food—and not "just enough," but really an abundance, as much as you want—is essential for recovery from diet culture. Being able to eat as many different kinds of food as you like, in whatever amounts you need to feel completely satisfied, allows your body to trust you again.

In my work with hundreds of clients, and in my own recovery from diet culture, I've found that pretty much *everyone* who struggles in their relationship with food doesn't allow themselves to have enough—even the folks who binge, who see themselves as eating "too much." The reality is that anyone who binges is *also* restricting, because we live in diet culture, and it would be impossible *not* to start thinking restrictive thoughts or engaging in restrictive behaviors as a response to bingeing. So even if the bingeing began for reasons unconnected to diet culture—as a response to childhood trauma, say—eventually (and often immediately) people feel pressured to diet in order to "make up for" having binged, and therefore they start restricting, too, even as the bingeing continues. The restricting just makes the bingeing worse.

For most people, though, bingeing starts precisely *because* of restriction—it's the Restriction Pendulum at work again, where bingeing is a natural response to dieting or "watching it" or "eating clean" or "being healthy" or whatever you want to call it. The pendulum has to swing back because you've been physically and psychologically deprived of food. When you're skimping on portions, restricting certain foods, berating yourself for what and how much you eat, and living under a regime of deprivation, the body's natural response is to eat as much as it can at any opportunity. Even if you feel like you're eating "too much," it's actually because you're not allowing yourself (both physically and mentally) to have *enough*.

Consider the case of my client Donna, who came to me because she was feeling out of control around food. She had episodes that she identified as emotional eating at least once a week, and she also often ate to the point of discomfort (though not outright binges) at dinner. Donna was in a larger body, and she blamed both her size and her eating on a lack of willpower.

Through our work together, Donna realized that willpower had nothing to do with it. Instead, most of the time she was physically and mentally restricting herself by eating only small portion sizes and sticking to a rigid list of foods she deemed "healthy" (which really meant dry, bland, and unsatisfying). On a day-to-day basis she wasn't allowing herself to have enough — enough variety, enough pleasure, enough food in general — and that scarcity was leading her to eat what she perceived as "too much" in her emotional-eating episodes. As she worked on letting go of this restrictive mind-set and replacing it with permission to eat in a way that felt truly satisfying, those episodes became rare occurrences, and she was able to recognize they'd been triggered by not eating enough. Confident that she was allowed to eat enough to feel satisfied both earlier in the day and in the evening, Donna stopped feeling uncomfortably full after dinner. Her body started trusting that it had — and would continue to have — enough.

Like Donna, the majority of my clients come to me because they *think* they have a problem with eating too much, with lack of willpower, with excess. They come to me wanting to develop a better connection with their fullness cues so they can stop eating when they're comfortably full, and wanting to find methods of coping with their emotions other than by eating. I always tell them that I can definitely help them with these goals, but that this can't be the place we start. Because truly, focusing on fullness and emotional eating is putting the cart before the horse.

The reason people eat to the point of discomfort is *not* because they're weak or greedy or emotionally broken; it's because they don't have enough, and because they don't trust that food will always be there when they want it. We can't stop at the point of fullness when we don't know how to honor our hunger — how to respond to it when it first pipes up rather than letting it build to a screaming emergency, or letting it scream for so long that its voice eventually becomes inaudible. In fact, when we aren't heeding our hunger signals (because of diet culture or any other reason), our bodies are programmed to start pumping out more and more of the hormones and neurotransmitters that drive us to eat — and that process virtually *guarantees* we'll feel out of control with food.[2] Moreover, we can't learn to use things other than food to cope with our feelings if those feelings are largely driven by *needing food*. Granted, once we release the restrictive thoughts and behaviors, we may also see that we need to develop some additional coping skills. But we can't know that for sure until we've recovered from the trauma of deprivation, which makes anyone reach for food to cope.

Focusing primarily on fullness and emotional eating instead of on eating *enough* keeps you stuck in diet culture—and therefore at war with food and your body. Diet culture demonizes eating emotionally and eating to the point of discomfort because it tells us these things will make us fat, and that fat is bad. If we accept that premise and try to address fullness and emotional eating without first making sure we have *enough*, we keep ourselves stuck under the Life Thief's thumb. We won't be able to solve our perceived eating problems because we're still caught up in the mind-set that created them.

To borrow another phrase from Audre Lorde, diet culture's tools will never dismantle diet culture's house. So when you're trying to relearn intuitive eating, the focus *must* be on finding ways to reassure your body and your brain that you have access to an abundance of food; that you won't be deprived again; and that you have true, unconditional permission to eat whatever you desire whenever you desire it. (By the way, intuitive eating does *not* mean "You're allowed to eat only when you're hungry, and you *must* stop when you're full." That's just another diet— the Hunger and Fullness Diet, as health coach Isabel Foxen Duke calls it—with restrictive rules, namely LISTEN TO YOUR BODY OR ELSE. More on that shortly.)

What if you can't hear your hunger cues at all? That means your body needs even *more* TLC, even *more* consistent eating, to recover from the deprivation that was imposed upon it. It means your body was so deprived that it basically stopped trying to get its needs met, like a neglected child who knows their cries won't be heard. If you've had significantly disordered eating or been dieting for a long time, you also might feel artificially full after only a few bites (an issue common to people with anorexia nervosa and other restrictive-eating disorders—which, don't forget, can affect folks of any weight). This is why people with active eating disorders should never attempt to jump straight into eating according to their hunger and fullness cues: those cues are going to be particularly out of whack, and will likely lead to restrictive-eating behaviors that only worsen the disorder.

Down the line, once you've truly healed from whatever level of deprivation you've experienced, you'll be able to trust your body's signals of hunger and fullness. Early on, though, the most important thing is simply to focus on breaking free from all forms of restriction, and learning to notice the ways your body might be telling you it needs food. The solution to wonky or absent hunger cues is showing your body that it won't be deprived anymore; that means eating consistent meals and snacks, even if you don't feel hungry. For people with active eating disorders, it also means working with an eating-disorder-savvy treatment team, including a psychotherapist and dietitian, who can support you through the process. Slowly, you'll start to rebuild that trust with your body. And eventually you'll get back to being able to recognize and honor your hunger the way you were *born* doing.

Reconnecting with Hunger

If you *are* in a place to start reconnecting with your hunger signals (or if you have the support of an experienced treatment team to work through this with you), here's an experiment to try:

First, pay attention to whether you experience any of these symptoms throughout the day:

- Difficulty making decisions
- Feeling irritable or annoyed
- Losing focus
- Bad breath or weird taste in your mouth
- Burping or gas
- Heartburn or acid reflux
- Feeling increasingly restless, uncomfortable, or agitated
- Thinking about food; fantasizing about your next meal or what to cook for dinner
- Fatigue or listlessness
- Sweating (without exerting yourself or being in a hot place)
- Headaches
- Nausea
- Ringing in the ears
- Anxiety or panic

If and when you notice any of these symptoms, try eating a satisfying snack or a meal (*not* diet food or a diet-size portion), and observe whether the symptoms diminish. If so, that particular symptom or set of symptoms may be one of the ways your body expresses hunger. Sensations of growling or gurgling in the stomach are just a few of many possible signs of hunger, and you may not feel these more "typical," stomach-related hunger sensations consistently if you have a history of dieting (aka disordered eating, aka following the Wellness Diet). For many people, if their stomachs do growl, it means their hunger is at a very high level—and that they missed some subtle signs before it reached that state. The symptoms listed above can all be signs of hunger, and some—including nausea, headaches, and sweating—may point to extreme hunger. Of course, these symptoms can also have causes unrelated to hunger; but if you notice that the symptoms respond positively to eating, or if you experience them only when it's been a couple of hours or more since you last ate, they're probably happening because you're hungry (even if you don't *think* you could/should be hungry).

These also aren't the only possible symptoms of hunger, so you might try this experiment with any other symptoms you experience regularly, and see if eating helps. One of my online course participants, for example, found that salivating is one of her hunger signals. Over time, you can learn the particular cues your body might be giving you that it's time to eat—just as parents learn to recognize their babies' and children's specific cries or other behaviors indicating hunger.

Your hunger signals are also likely to shift as time goes on, just as children's expressions of hunger evolve as they grow up— from wailing as babies, to a few words as toddlers, to a clear "I'm hungry" as elementary-school kids, to just opening the fridge and making themselves some food as preteens and adolescents. Once you're well versed in noticing and responding to the various hunger signals your body gives you, you probably won't need to think about them as much. For example, having relearned intuitive eating about ten years ago, I no longer have to consciously scan my body for signs of hunger. Instead I'm struck with an awareness that I'm hungry, and to what degree ("snack-hungry," for example, or "meal-hungry"); I then go looking for food as soon as possible. I intuitively recognize my hunger, and I trust that I'm allowed to eat as much food as it takes to satisfy it. The same is true for intuitive eaters of all shapes, sizes, and identities.

We might experience other shifts in our hunger signals throughout our life spans. For example, we could become pregnant, go through menopause, or undergo a gender transition— all of which shift our bodies' hormone levels and hunger cues. Certain lifesaving medications, such as cancer drugs or anti-depressants, can likewise alter our appetites. Whatever changes we go through in our lives, though, we can experiment and figure out our body's particular ways of asking us to feed it. Intuitive eating during pregnancy or cancer treatment will probably feel different than intuitive eating without those conditions. But intuitive eating is not about experiencing "perfect" hunger signals that never change—it's about doing your best in any circumstance to honor your body's need for food without letting diet-culture beliefs get in the way.

Not only is it important to honor the signals that your body needs food, it's essential to feed yourself at regular intervals—and to feed yourself *enough*—even if your body isn't giving you clear hunger signals. That's why intuitive eating differs radically from the Hunger and Fullness Diet (including the "hunger-directed-eating" diet that's currently having a moment). Intuitive eating isn't just about tuning in to your body, although that's certainly part of it. It's also about eating when you're *not* hungry because you're about to go into a long meeting with no food and you know you'll get the shakes if you don't have lunch first—aka eating for self-care. It's also about having some cake at your friend's birthday party because you like the taste and you want to celebrate—aka eating for pleasure. And it's about honoring that little voice in your head saying "I need more," even when you think you "should" be full. (As discussed with the Restriction Pendulum, you may continue needing more for a good long while after a period of restriction before things even out.) You're allowed to eat both when your body is giving you hunger signals and when it's not. You're allowed to eat at parties or on dates even if you're not particularly hungry. You're allowed to eat when you've had a hard day. *You are allowed to eat for any reason you freaking well feel like it, anytime you want.*

Does that mean you'll be eating more in response to food advertising and large portion sizes at restaurants? No—quite the opposite. A 2017 review of the scientific research on how chronic dieting affects food consumption found that not only do dieters eat more in response to food-related advertisements or large portion sizes, they also eat more of both high-fat foods *and* foods labeled as *healthy* or *low-calorie,* even if those labels are false.[3] Dieters, in other words, are highly susceptible to both food-industry and diet-industry marketing.

Nondieters, by contrast, aren't swayed by advertising or portion sizes; they tend to eat similar amounts when exposed to these things as they do otherwise, because they're driven by internal rather than external cues. (You may have heard differently in years past thanks to some buzzy findings by food-marketing researcher Brian Wansink, who is largely responsible for the widespread belief that people eat more in response to larger portion sizes. But Wansink's research has since been thoroughly discredited, and in 2018 he resigned in disgrace from his post at Cornell University.[4]) Dieters are susceptible to external pressure to eat because chronic deprivation makes them hyperaware of food-related stimuli in their environment, whereas nondieters tend to filter out those stimuli. All the din about food and dieting becomes white noise when you aren't trying to restrain your eating. So instead of pushing initiatives aimed at trying to reduce restaurant portion sizes or curb food-industry marketing, public-health officials who worry about the influence of environmental cues on our food intake would be much better off working to end chronic dieting.

Moreover, as we've been discussing, our so-called "emotional" reasons for eating often diminish or disappear when we eat enough. As one of the participants in my intuitive eating online course revealed: "I'm not an emotional eater—how's that for an aha moment? All this time, I thought I was 'sick in the head,' as my mama would say. But NO, I was freaking starving. All those years of running kids around, hauling groceries, playing tennis, cleaning house—then trying to survive on [too little food] for breakfast and lunch. No wonder I was like a fiend by three o'clock in the afternoon!" Her observation illustrates how we can convince ourselves we eat for emotional reasons, when in fact it's simply because we're hungry—and we just didn't recognize the signs. That's all the more reason to start trusting the inner voice telling us to eat, rather than second-guessing it.

The Stray-Cat Effect

When I was about four years old, a gray kitten took up residence under some bushes in our yard. Clearly a stray, she was so timid that she wouldn't come near us at first. But my mom and I put out food for her every day, and slowly she started to peek her head out and look at us as we approached. Eventually the kitten began coming out when we brought the food, then sniffing our hands and letting us pet her. Finally my mom caught her and brought her inside—at which point, of course, the kitten freaked out and had to get used to us and her surroundings all over again.

We had to be incredibly gentle with her, giving her tons of time and space to adjust, and she remained quite timid for the rest of her life (about seventeen more years). She'd clearly gone through a lot in her months as a stray that stayed with her in a deep way. Instead of walking around like she owned the place and jumping up wherever she wanted to sit, as most cats do, she'd place a paw on your leg, with a look as if to say, "Is this OK? Can I sit in your lap? Will you pet me?" We had to reassure her all the time, but she was the sweetest cat I've ever had, and I've had some sweeties over the years.

When it comes to recovering from diet culture, your body and brain are like that stray cat. You might need a long time to work up the courage to stop dieting, then even longer to adjust to life without diet rules. You might feel like a scared baby animal that's gone through a lot of trauma, because that's what it is.

"Diet culture is trauma in and of itself," explains Lilia Graue, a marriage and family therapist and medical doctor who specializes in recovery from disordered eating. "It threatens our most basic need, which is the need to belong. You're bombarded by messages of 'Your body is wrong,' 'Your body doesn't belong,' 'Your body doesn't conform to what we think is worthy or lovable or acceptable.' How can you not be traumatized by that?"

The word *trauma* means an experience of overwhelming stress. And when you think about the levels of stress we experience from living in diet culture, it's clear that trauma is exactly what we're dealing with. Just like any other oppressive system, diet culture is traumatic.

Another form of trauma that diet culture imposes on us is food deprivation, which not only triggers the out-of-control swings of the Restriction Pendulum but increases cortisol levels[5]—a physiological reaction to stress seen in other forms of trauma, including weight-based discrimination. When you're recovering from diet culture, you need to treat yourself kindly and gently in order to heal from these distressing experiences. You need to reassure yourself constantly, to let yourself know that everything is OK. Your body and brain are going to ask you for reassurance in a million different ways: "Can I eat now?" "Am I going to get enough?" "Are you sure?" Your job is to continue telling yourself that yes, there is enough, and yes, you're allowed to eat as much as you want. You must be truly compassionate with yourself. I know that's hard, but think of how you'd comfort a scared pet or an anxious child—in your best moments, you would never yell at them or do anything to reinforce their fear, right? (I say "best moments" because of course we all have our snippy ones, too.) Instead you'd work to comfort them, over and over again—and that's exactly what you have to do with your brain and your body in recovery from diet culture.

Remember the Minnesota Starvation Experiment from Chapter 6? The participants in that study struggled to restore their relationships with food long after the experiment was over, in a way that illustrates how traumatic even short-term food restriction can be. Many of the men in the study reported consistently eating to the point of discomfort after they left the trial; one man described the feeling of persistent hunger after the experiment as a "year-long cavity" that needed to be filled.[6] The men's estimates of how long it took them to recover from the ordeal ranged from a few months to two years—and this was after a "semi-starvation" period that lasted only *six months*. Meanwhile, dieters in our society go through these periods for years at a stretch or dozens of separate times, often over a span of decades.

So give yourself compassion for how long it takes to recover from the trauma of dieting, and allow for some ups and downs as you go through the process. Expect that your body might react to any ongoing threat of deprivation in ways that seem strange or disproportionate. I've had clients report bursting into tears when the grocery store was out of the cookies they craved, or bingeing on everything in sight because they'd waited a little too long before eating their afternoon snack. When you've been through a famine—which is essentially what dieting is—your body will have a hair-trigger response to any sign of not getting its needs met for a while. It's like that stray kitten, or any other skittish animal: it needs some TLC, some consistent reassurance that you're not going to deprive it again.

Above all, don't shame yourself for having needs—or for not knowing exactly what they are right now. Relearning intuitive eating is like any learning experience: it's going to be messy and awkward, but eventually you'll get more practiced at it, and things will start to come more easily in time. Eventually the urgency and frequency of your thoughts about food will dissipate, and it will become much easier to tell when you're hungry—and what you're in the mood to eat.

You also deserve support through this process. Some discomfort is normal when you're giving up dieting, but it's always helpful to have a community of people who are on the same path and can listen and commiserate with you about the ups and downs. And if you're experiencing anxiety about food and body image that's interfering with your day-to-day life, reach out and get help. Take a look at the Resources section at the back of the book for recommendations of professionals trained in intuitive eating and diet-culture recovery, and see Chapter 11 for advice on building community support.

What If There's Really Not Enough?

If you're living in poverty and don't have enough to eat as a result, what does that mean for your ability to overcome deprivation and make peace with food? Unfortunately, it just makes it that much harder, and you're not alone in struggling with this issue. Food insecurity affects how millions of people relate to food. "I grew up really, really poor, and food insecurity was a real part of my day-to-day life," says Ijeoma Oluo, now a writer who covers race and social-justice issues. "So I always had this kind of grasping, desperate relationship with food." Critics of intuitive eating often rightfully point out that it can sometimes feel a bit classist because some of the solutions that it offers assume there's enough food available to keep things you love in stock, and that there's money to buy new clothes if and when your body size changes. This is one of the many reasons why preventing and treating disordered eating isn't just an individual issue—it's a systemic one, requiring solutions that go way beyond telling people how to eat or what to choose at the grocery store.

If you don't have the means to afford food in a consistent way, there are definite limitations on how much you can do to make peace with food, because that constant sense of deprivation is going to interfere with your ability to trust that there's *enough* (and with your sense of peace in general). Food insecurity is a form of ongoing trauma, and the outcome is the same as dieting in the sense that it gets you swinging on the Restriction Pendulum, where very real deprivation drives you to eat *all the food right now* as soon as you do have access to food, because you don't know when you'll be able to buy it again. "We would have times where we had absolutely nothing, and then on the first of the month we'd go shopping," Oluo says. "We just tried to eat as much as possible because we had food. You get this 'I have to eat it all now' feeling."

This is a common experience, and it's reflected in the emerging research on the connection between food insecurity and disordered eating. A 2017 study of a low-income population in urban San Antonio, for instance, found that food insecurity is associated with significant levels of rebound eating, with more than 56 percent of participants reporting binge eating, overeating, or night eating.[7] The risk of these issues increases with rising levels of deprivation, and 17 percent of people with the most severe food insecurity were found to meet *clinical criteria* for an eating disorder—far higher than the single-digit rates of clinically diagnosed eating disorders in the general population. This shows that the stereotypical view of eating disorders as a disease of wealthy white folks is sorely mistaken; most of the participants in this study were Latinx and black people living far below the poverty line.

Food insecurity and diet culture don't exist in separate silos, either: the same study found that those with the greatest degree of food insecurity also had the highest levels of internalized weight stigma, as well as the highest levels of bulimic behaviors and overexercising as a way to compensate for eating. (Those last two findings surprised even the researchers, who had expected not to find compensatory behaviors in this highly food-insecure population.) So even if binge eating begins in response to food insecurity rather than concerns about weight and shape, it's clear that diet-culture beliefs about body size also come into play for those who lack reliable access to food. The increasing pressure on this population to use food-assistance dollars for "healthy" food rather than "junk" food is another example of how diet culture is infiltrating the conversation about food insecurity and piling more stigma on an already marginalized group.

The nexus of food insecurity and disordered eating is complicated—and inadequately understood. I don't have all the answers, but I do know this: we need to make a lot of changes at the collective level to help stop the cycle of poverty that keeps people stuck in food insecurity—not just because of how it affects people's relationships with food, but because it's a matter of social justice. And for anyone trying to heal from disordered eating—regardless of race, gender, income, or education level—the most important thing is having *enough* to eat on a continual basis. So instead of trying to curtail access to foods deemed "unhealthy" in low-income communities, limiting what people are able to buy with their food-assistance dollars, and engaging in "anti-obesity" campaigns that serve only to reinforce weight stigma, we as a society need to work on ensuring that everyone has reliable, consistent access to food. We need to stop pathologizing convenience foods and "overeating," because sometimes those things are essential for people's survival. And we need to burn diet culture to the ground, because when people living in extreme poverty and hunger feel the need to use disordered behaviors to compensate for the food that's keeping them alive, there's something deeply wrong in the world.

A Word About Fullness

As I've alluded to throughout this chapter, stopping eating in response to fullness really tends to fall into place once you get the hang of honoring your body's needs for food, and once you trust that you'll always have *enough*—both enough food in general, and enough variety and pleasure in your food choices. You need to trust that you're allowed to eat as much as you want of the foods you desire, anytime. Part of what keeps people eating past the point of comfortable fullness is the belief that their food is going to be taken away or placed off-limits again, so they have to get it all in now while they can. So if you want to be able to honor your fullness and stop before getting painfully full, you have to focus on *allowance*—allowing yourself to eat consistently throughout the day, and allowing yourself access to all foods, rather than making certain things verboten.

What do I mean by "all foods," you might ask. We'll explore that next.

CHAPTER 9

Stop Labeling Food as *Good* or *Bad*

Here's a quiz to gauge your stage of letting go of diet-culture thinking: Which is a better food choice, an apple or a burger?

If you picked the apple, that's totally understandable coming from diet culture. One of its hallmarks is demonizing some foods while elevating others, and at this point in history the foods it tends to elevate are so-called "whole" foods such as apples. Things like burgers—particularly the fast-food varieties— are the ones that get demonized. The "processed" meat (or vegetable protein), the carbs in the bun, and the corn syrup in the ketchup are all points of contention for the Wellness Diet.

In reality, though, the answer to which of these two foods is "better" is *neither*. The burger and the apple are equal in moral value—in that neither of them has one. One is not even categorically "better" than the other in a nutritional sense, although each of them might be more helpful for different purposes. For example, the apple is crunchy, refreshing, and full of fiber. If you're in the mood for something sweet, you'd be better off with the apple (or a cookie, or some candy), but it's certainly *not* a satisfying choice if what you really need is a sustaining meal. The burger makes a lot more sense for that purpose, and it's also comforting, delicious, and full of important nutrients— plus it's affordable and convenient, if we're talking about a fast-food version. These foods have different breakdowns of micronutrients (vitamins and minerals) and macronutrients (carbs, protein, and fat), and your body needs all of them. You literally cannot live on fruits and vegetables alone.

The Wellness Diet has turned nutrition and health into moral battlegrounds, but that has led only to increased stigma and therefore increased health risks—greater, in fact, than the risks people might incur by eating the very foods that diet culture demonizes.[1] As we've been discussing, the more that people are subjected to moralized views about food and health, the worse their health becomes. Foods aren't inherently "healthy" or "unhealthy"; when we judge them as such, we're looking at them only through the Life Thief's lens (which, may I remind you, is a racist, sexist, body-negative one). Life beyond diet culture is about having variety and balance in your food choices, and about getting your needs met, both for nutrients *and for satisfaction and pleasure.*

That's why one of the key tenets of intuitive eating is that there's no such thing as "good" or "bad" food. This thinking flies in the face of everything diet culture teaches us about food. Yet when you destigmatize foods and look at them all as equally worthy options, it takes away the irresistible pull toward "forbidden" foods (don't those always taste the sweetest?). Instead, you're able to choose what you *truly* want and need in any given moment. Refusing to follow diet culture's rules about "good" and "bad" foods gives you back the power and the agency to make your own decisions about what to eat. It removes the physical and emotional deprivation that go along with "being good" by diet culture's standards. It restores your autonomy.

As discussed throughout this book, truly holistic well-being is about much more than the purely physical dimension—that is, the one privileged by the Wellness Diet when it talks about "holistic" health. Sure, eating *only* burgers probably wouldn't be the most health-promoting thing to do in the long run, but neither would eating only apples—or eating only "whole" foods, for that matter, because that puts you at risk of orthorexia, with all of its negative mental- and physical-health outcomes. That's not to shame anyone for subsisting primarily on one type of food; if the only sustenance you have access to is burgers, for example, that's certainly better than the alternative of no food at all. But in situations where you have access to (and can afford) more variety, any severely limited menu is likely to harm your overall well-being. Truly holistic health encompasses physical, mental, emotional, and social aspects—including freedom from stigma, reliable access to food and shelter, and sufficient resources for transportation, childcare, and medical care, as well as the right to pleasure and satisfaction in your life as a whole, including your food. Truly holistic health is about so much more than what you eat.

Thus, making peace with all kinds of foods, even the formerly "forbidden" ones, supports your mental and emotional health as well as your physical well-being. Research has shown that intuitive eaters, who don't have any "off-limits" foods or follow any diet-culture rules, have better health outcomes on an impressive array of measures: lower cardiovascular risk, decreased triglyceride levels, more-favorable levels of HDL cholesterol, lower rates of disordered eating, less likelihood of feeling out of control with food, less food-related anxiety, less internalization of the thin ideal, lower levels of body dissatisfaction and shame, greater enjoyment of food, increased body appreciation, less self-silencing behavior, higher sensitivity to their own internal states, higher levels of self-compassion, greater life satisfaction, more proactive coping skills, and better self-esteem.[2] People don't drop dead when they let go of diet culture's rules, tune in to their bodies' cues and desires, and figure out what they enjoy eating. On the contrary, they *increase* their chances of having positive health outcomes. Not restricting or feeling guilty about food means you free yourself from emotional and physical deprivation. You get off the Restriction Pendulum and find peace.

The Pleasure Principle and the "Honeymoon Phase"

Have you ever had the craving for a food that diet culture demonizes—say, a cupcake—and opted for a "lite" or Wellness Diet–approved version instead, because that's what you thought you "should" do? Odds are it didn't float your boat, because what you wanted was the real thing—sugar, butter, flour, and all. And what happened then? Maybe you just suffered in silence, pretending the sorry substitute was good enough. Or maybe you've trained yourself over a long-enough period of dieting to *almost* believe you prefer diet culture's version. Often, though, you can't quite fool yourself; your brain is too smart and knows it's been cheated. Dates and unsweetened cocoa powder do not a cupcake make. At that point, you might end up eating a bunch of other things in search of the satisfaction you were after— perhaps eventually including the "forbidden" dessert you'd wanted from the start.

What would it feel like if you no longer had to bother with these kinds of substitutions? To just eat the cupcake in the first place? When you're the one making your own food choices (rather than having diet culture pulling the strings), you can choose the thing you really want, enjoy it without guilt or self-loathing, then move on with your life.

Taking pleasure in food is a central force in intuitive eating: rather than trying to talk yourself out of your desires for so-called "forbidden" foods, you give yourself full, unconditional permission to enjoy them—along with every other kind of food—as often as you like. You're able to seek out and find satisfying things to eat, instead of trying to convince yourself you enjoy the things you're forcing yourself to eat. Savoring food becomes an everyday experience—not something reserved for weekends or "cheat days"—so you never have to panic that you're not going to be "allowed" to have any more of your favorite snack once this bag is gone. It's here for you again whenever you want.

Of course, we all have to pay attention to details such as our budgets, which foods are available in any given moment, and what's going to keep us energized through the long meeting or the dance party. For people with low incomes, certain foods may not be available regularly. No matter what your circumstances, though, you're allowed to make pleasure a driving force in your food choices, and you don't have to feel guilty about that. Intuitive eating is all about taking your *desires* into account with every meal or snack, even when you're factoring in how hungry you are, what you can afford, or what your schedule looks like that day. You're certainly not going to end up in a perfectly blissful state of satisfaction every time you eat—or even know exactly what you want in a given moment, especially when you're just starting the process of making peace with food. But in doing the best you can to choose foods that give you pleasure, you'll be more satisfied over the long term than you ever would be by following diet culture's rules.

One of the biggest worries I hear from people when they start thinking about prioritizing pleasure over diet culture's rules is this: *What if I never eat anything but brownies again?* That concern is understandable, but I can assure you that if you do have a brownies-only moment, it won't last long. People relearning intuitive eating often go through a "Honeymoon Phase": when you've been restricted for a while from eating certain foods, you're going to reach a point where those foods are all you want. It's like you're at the beginning of a new relationship with them where you can't get enough, and nothing else seems

appealing (much like the Honeymoon Phase with a new romantic partner). This is a common part of the process. Remember
the Restriction Pendulum, where you go from restricting food
to eating *all* the food? The Honeymoon Phase is similar: you go
from restricting *particular* foods to having intense cravings for
and eating larger amounts of those foods—namely, the ones
you've been deprived of.

It doesn't mean there's anything wrong with you. On the
contrary, it's to be expected when you've been dieting. For example, a 2005 study found that women who were deprived of chocolate for a week experienced greater cravings for chocolate, and
increased their consumption of chocolaty foods when the deprivation period ended—and this reaction was significantly stronger among people who were "restrained" eaters, aka chronic
dieters.[3] In that study, dieters also reported more frequent food
cravings in general than did unrestrained eaters. Not that
there's anything wrong with food cravings, of course—but the
operative factor here is the deprivation. People who deprive
themselves end up having *more* cravings than people who honor
their cravings, and they are likelier to go through a Honeymoon
Phase with particular foods.

The Honeymoon Phase is highly disorienting, and it can be
tempting to restrict your access to particular foods again when
you find yourself going to town on them constantly. Trust me,
though: going through the Honeymoon Phase is a sign that you
need *more* permission with these foods, not less.* You might also

---

* As I've stressed throughout, if you have a genuine medical condition (rather
than one invented by diet culture) that makes certain foods anathema to
your body, there's no need to eat them to prove anything to yourself—and
you likely won't experience a Honeymoon Phase with those foods anyway.
Your Honeymoon Phase is much likelier to involve foods that were "forbidden" for diet-culture reasons (including Wellness Diet reasons, as discussed
in Chapters 2 and 3) than it is to center around foods that your body truly

need the help of a therapist, dietitian, recovery coach, or other anti-diet support person as you weather this period because, as I said, it can throw you for a loop. (See the Resources section at the back of the book for recommendations on how to find someone to work with.) You can also work on making peace with previously off-limits foods one at a time, in a systematic way, to make it feel safer (again, perhaps with the help of one of those anti-diet support people). Ultimately, however you approach it, know that allowing yourself to take pleasure in the foods you once forbade yourself—and to truly believe that you're allowed to eat and enjoy *all* foods—is the key to moving through the Honeymoon Phase. Eventually you'll show your body that these foods won't be made off-limits again, and then you'll naturally start wanting a greater variety of foods.

I can't cite an exact timeline for how long that will take. Folks subjected to the trauma of deprivation for longer periods of time often take longer to recover from it, but sometimes people get to such a point of having had *enough* that something snaps and they give up dieting relatively quickly. I've spoken to dozens of people in both camps, and dozens more who fall somewhere in between. No matter how long it takes for you, though, the key to moving through the Honeymoon Phase is to grant yourself unconditional permission to eat anything you desire. As all Honeymoon Phases do, it will eventually end.

---

cannot tolerate. People with serious reactions to a particular food don't usually *want* to eat it. Ultimately, though, your body is yours to do with as you wish: If you find yourself with a persistent craving for a food you're allergic to, you could technically decide to eat it if you want. As a human being with bodily autonomy, you have the ability to eat anything you desire that's available to you. Again, you probably wouldn't want to eat something that would send you to the hospital (nor am I saying you should), but just remembering that it's actually *your* decision can help any food-allergy restrictions feel less like diet rules and more like self-care.

This *doesn't* mean, by the way, that you'll never crave (or eat) those previously off-limits foods again. That's a misconception fomented by diet culture, but it's just another one of its lies. Moving past the Honeymoon Phase simply means you'll stop wanting the previously forbidden foods *all the time*, but you might still want them from time to time—perhaps even every day, but never in the frenzied way you desired them before. For example, at this point in my life I eat chips of some kind almost every day, but I'm not sneaking them, berating myself for eating them, or eating to the point of extreme discomfort (as I did when I viewed them as contraband). I also never restrict my eating for the rest of the day in response to having eaten them, and I eat a wide variety of other foods that I enjoy in addition to the chips. So it's not about getting the foods you fear off your menu. Instead, it's about getting them off your "off-limits" list, and giving yourself unfettered permission to eat them. Then, from that place, you're able to make choices about what you truly *desire*. There's something incredibly powerful about saying to yourself, "I have unconditional permission to eat whatever I want—so now what do I want?"

What About Nutrition?

The diet-culture message about nutrition goes something like this: if you're allowed to eat whatever you want, you're going to eat nothing but "unhealthy" foods—so you *need* food rules to keep you from eating yourself into an early grave. That's the rationale that drives people to keep seeking external nutrition advice, keep paying for expensive Wellness Diet programs, keep buying health magazines, and keep clicking on fearmongering nutrition headlines. And in diet culture, nutrition and pleasure really can *seem* diametrically opposed. Research shows that people who are less health-conscious when it comes to their food choices have higher levels of pleasure associated with food and eating, whereas those who are more health-conscious about what they eat find less pleasure in eating.[4]

In reality, though, pleasure and nutrition are highly correlated: The people who let themselves eat whatever they want, take pleasure in food, and *care less* about nutrition tend to have improved nutrient intake—and consume a greater variety of foods, a positive nutritional indicator—than dieters.[5] And even though in the Honeymoon Phase it might *feel* like you'll never stop eating previously forbidden foods, research has found that intuitive eating doesn't increase people's consumption of what diet culture dubs "junk food"; intuitive eaters and dieters actually eat the same amount of these fun foods.[6] Overall, then, intuitive eaters have more balance, more variety, and more pleasure in their eating. Dieters *worry* more about nutrition, but that doesn't translate into any nutritional benefit.

Granted, when you're in the Honeymoon Phase, it may seem like the day will never come when you think, "What I really want is a nice big serving of vegetables with this meal." In fact, in the Honeymoon Phase diet culture–approved foods such as veggies, fruits, and certain proteins may now seem like the "forbidden" ones. But when you get to the other side of the Honeymoon Phase, *nothing* is off-limits—not sweets or chips or "processed" foods, and not salads or kale or "whole" foods, either. When people settle into trusting that they're allowed to eat whatever they wish, they typically find they want a wide variety of foods—some savory and some sweet, some heartier and some more refreshing, some homemade and some "processed." If we can break the diet mentality, get back in touch with our bodies, and use our internal cues along with our sense of satisfaction and pleasure to guide our food choices, we're going to end up having balance and variety in our eating in a way that supports our overall well-being.

Even for diseases where food choices play an undeniable role in management—diabetes, heart disease, acid reflux—it's helpful not to treat any foods as "bad" or off-limits. Instead of saying, for example, "I'm not allowed to have certain foods because of my disease," you can say, "I'm allowed to eat anything I want, and I can *also* learn how those foods might affect my disease so that I can make informed choices."

Take diabetes, for example: diet culture makes people with this condition live in constant fear of carbohydrates, but these nutrients don't need to be off-limits at all—they just need to be understood. Yes, someone with diabetes might have a blood-sugar spike from eating a carbs-only meal or snack—within their rights as an autonomous human being, if that's what they want or need to do—but the likelihood of that spike significantly diminishes if the meal or snack also includes foods containing protein, fat, and fiber, since all of those nutrients help slow the digestion of carbs and thereby stabilize blood-sugar levels. So if you have diabetes, you can experiment with various food combinations and recipes—in addition to paying attention to your hunger cues, energy levels, and sense of satisfaction and pleasure in eating—to figure out what keeps your blood sugar in a range that works for you, while also allowing you to enjoy life. Instead of demonizing carbs, as diet culture would have everyone with diabetes do, you can learn to work with these nutrients.

In other cases, the "health" rationale for avoiding particular foods is purely a product of diet culture. There's no scientific validity to those color-coded tests that measure IgG antibodies and tell you that you're "sensitive" to a million different foods, just as there's no scientific validity to hair testing, cell testing, applied kinesiology (aka muscle testing), or a multitude of other bogus tests. Any benefit people feel from cutting out foods in response to those spurious tests likely stems from the "nocebo effect": when you're told that particular foods are causing you problems and you cut them out, it's normal to feel better temporarily simply thanks to the power of suggestion. Eventually, however, the stress and difficulty of eliminating the supposedly offending foods tend to outweigh any good feelings induced by the nocebo effect. So if you've had certain foods on your banned list because one of these bogus tests made you fear them, I invite you to consider bringing them back into your life—and working to make peace with them instead.

Sugar Panic and the Problem with Nutrition Science

"Sugar will kill you." That's one of the most persistent nutrition-related beliefs I hear these days. But is it really true? Not so much—and the problems with that belief speak to a larger issue about the way nutrition science is conducted.

First of all, most nutrition research you hear about *isn't* done in labs with a control group that gets one food while an experimental group gets another. That kind of rigorous research is expensive and hard to conduct. Keeping people's eating under a microscope long enough to get meaningful results demands a great deal of labor on the part of the researchers. It poses a major inconvenience for the study participants. Nobody's got time (or money) for that.

Most nutrition research is therefore instead done by asking groups of people about their eating habits, and about the health conditions they have now and any new ones they develop during follow-up periods. Sometimes the researchers draw blood or collect other samples, and sometimes they look at medical records; other times they merely have people self-report what happened. The researchers then divide the participants into categories based on how much of a given food or nutrient they consume. In most nutrition studies, it's five categories (known as quintiles), but sometimes it's four (called quartiles) or three (called tertiles). Researchers like using these groupings because they allow them to determine a relative risk of disease among groups of people with low, medium, or high consumption of a particular food or food group. While some statisticians believe this method can lead to inaccuracies and difficulty comparing results across studies, it remains fairly standard practice in nutrition studies and other population-level health research.[7] Nutrition researchers compare the people in the lowest quintile (or quartile, or tertile) to the people in the higher quintiles (or quartiles, or tertiles), examining which health outcomes occur in the people who consume more of a certain food or nutrient versus the ones who eat less, as in: Were the people who reported eating more vegetables more or less likely to have a heart attack five years later? What about the people who reported eating more fats? And so on.

In recent years, a few studies have indicated that people in the lowest quintile of consumption of added sugars have a lower risk of heart disease than the people in the higher quintiles. That science is still controversial, however.[8] Yet the existence of even *some* evidence suggesting that eating sugar raises heart risk justifies cutting out sugar, right? Not so fast. What we really need to know is this: What exactly are the cutoff points for each of the quintiles in the studies? Those numbers matter. The way the general public (and even some health professionals) interpret this emerging science, it's as if everyone in the lowest quintile of sugar consumption was eating *zero* sugar. But that's not the case at all. In fact, according to the evidence we have to date linking sugar with cardiovascular disease, the people in the quintile with the lowest added-sugar consumption (who, remember, have the *lowest* risk of getting or dying from heart disease) consume an amount of added sugar equivalent to eating some sweetened foods at every meal and every snack, *and* having dessert every day.

For example, you could have some fruit-on-the-bottom yogurt with sweetened granola at breakfast, a nice big sandwich with honey mustard on sweetened bread at lunch, honey-roasted nuts or sugar-added trail mix for a snack, a sweetened salad dressing as part of your dinner, and a regular-size candy bar or giant bakery cookie for dessert, and still be in the lowest quintile of consumption for added sugar, with the lowest heart risk.[9] Meanwhile, the people in the highest quintile of added-sugar intake consume the equivalent of *at least* 7.5 regular-size candy bars *every single day*. If someone is eating that way on a daily basis, it's a good bet something's going on in their life and their relationship with food.

This is not to food-shame anyone, by any means. It's simply to say that if you're consuming as much sugar on the reg as the people in the highest quintile, you have your reasons. Maybe an eating disorder or a history of chronic dieting is causing you to binge eat, for example. (Shockingly, nutrition studies don't typically ask participants about their disordered-eating behaviors, nor do they control for them in any way.[10]) Another reason might be weight stigma, which has been linked with higher consumption of sugary foods (because, as we've seen, trying to shame people into eating by diet culture's rules tends to result in their doing the exact opposite).[11] People who experience greater weight stigma in their everyday lives are more likely to consume sugar-sweetened drinks and fast food. Not only that, but people subjected to weight-stigmatizing language in an experimental setting have been shown to eat more than twice as many sweets as nonstigmatized controls.

Eating disorders, chronic dieting, and weight stigma can all therefore lead to greater sugar intake (and these conditions are all *independently* associated with an increased risk of cardiovascular problems).[12] In other words, the increased heart risk for people in the highest quintile of sugar consumption might have nothing to do with sugar itself—and everything to do with an underlying condition that happens to make them eat more sugar.

One thing *not* driving people to eat more sugar, by the way, is "addiction." Food isn't the addictive substance that diet culture makes it out to be—and that goes for foods high in added sugar just as much as for any other type of food. A 2016 review of the scientific literature found no convincing evidence in humans to support the belief that sugar is addictive.[13] Findings from animal studies (which can't be used to make any sort of claim about what happens in humans, and can only be used to guide further research *on* humans) indicate that any addiction-like behaviors around sugar occur only when the animals have intermittent access to sugar—*not* when they're allowed to eat as much of it as they want at any time. Only when the animals are periodically *deprived* of sugar do they eat in a way that might look or feel "addictive." The deprivation—not any chemical properties of the food itself—drives their bingeing. And whereas proponents of "sugar addiction" theory love to point out that "processed" food is engineered to achieve a perfect "bliss point" of sweetness that makes it supposedly irresistible to the reward centers in our brains, research has in fact shown that *only dieters* experience significant activation of brain regions associated with reward in response to sweet foods.[14] The brains of nondieters, by contrast, seem to remain relatively unfazed by sugar.

These issues with sugar research apply to nutrition science as a whole.

First, animal studies cannot be extrapolated to humans; at best, they can alert researchers to areas for further scientific study *on* humans. Those human studies, in turn, must be repeated multiple times with large groups of people in well-designed experiments (that is, in randomized, controlled trials). Only if those results are replicated across multiple studies can we begin to use them to guide human behavior.

Second, whenever you see a report linking a certain food

with some negative health outcome, that doesn't mean the food *causes* the outcome. As I've emphasized throughout this book, correlation is not causation. And you can bet that the people in the lowest quintile or quartile of consumption of that particular food still eat quite a bit of it, on average. They're not ascetics who avoid that food at all costs—and you needn't be one, either.

That's the main point I want to convey in this discussion of nutrition research: there's no scientific justification for demonizing and cutting out whole categories of foods, the way the Wellness Diet tells you to. Trying to do that usually backfires: you end up bingeing on or feeling "addicted" to those foods when you gain access to them again. Ironically, once you break free of diet culture's rules, heal from the trauma of food deprivation, and start following your own inner wisdom about what to eat, you're much likelier to end up in good health than those who obsess about nutrition. You'll find yourself naturally relaxing around the foods that diet culture demonizes. You may even stop wanting to eat as much of them as a result—not because you consider them "bad" in any way, but simply because you know you can enjoy them anytime, and you have lots of other foods you enjoy, too.

Consider the Source

When I was deep in disordered-eating and orthorexic attitudes about food, I worked as a journalist covering food, nutrition, and health for major national publications. In my role as an editor, I encouraged writers to include scaremongering statements about how the "obesity epidemic" was supposedly going to make this generation of kids die before their parents (a claim based on false assumptions and *no* statistical analysis, yet cited by more than 1,000 academic papers and countless health and nutrition publications[15]). When I wrote food-and-nutrition articles of my own, my editors usually let my food-shaming statements stand — including insinuations that gluten was the devil, catty asides about corn syrup, and cringeworthy headlines such as "How to Avoid Airport Fare" and "Soul Food: Not So Good for the Body." When I pitched stories fueled by my own orthorexic curiosity about how to be "healthier," I was rewarded with bylines, paychecks, and praise from my editors.

I wasn't the only journalist fanning the flames of the Wellness Diet, of course. I'd guess that most reporters and editors covering food and nutrition are caught up in diet-culture thinking, just like the majority of the population in Western society. That's vital to keep in mind whenever you read articles about nutrition and health. The people in charge of those magazines and newspapers and blogs are as human as anyone else — and, in my experience, often even *more* likely to be influenced by diet-culture beliefs: not only are they exposed to so much of it at work, but a certain proportion of them start on this career path because of their own obsessions and insecurities about food and health (as I did). Nutrition media consistently reinforces diet culture–driven ideas about "good" and "bad" foods, but that's not because those ideas are The Truth — it's because members of the media believe them, and therefore don't question them.

That goes for nutrition scientists as well. Instead of looking at study participants in terms of *truly* holistic measures of health — their relationship with food, their life circumstances, the forces driving their eating behaviors — nutrition researchers look at food as the primary, and often the only, independent variable. That's certainly understandable, given how diet culture perpetuates the myth that "you are what you eat," and given that most people who go into the field of nutrition have bought into that belief. (I also say this as someone who went back to school to become a dietitian because of my own fierce belief in many tenets of the Wellness Diet at the time.) Scientists are people, too, and in general the people who conduct nutrition science are invested in the idea that nutrition is an important—if not *the most* important—determinant of health.

Unfortunately, that point of view excludes quite a few factors that have more influence over health outcomes than what you eat: weight stigma and other forms of discrimination; poverty; food and job insecurity; traumatic experiences; relational difficulties; and disordered eating, to name just a few. All of these factors are effectively erased in the overwhelming majority of scientific literature on nutrition, which can make it seem like food alone is responsible for health disparities, reinforcing the diet-culture beliefs about food that most people in our society already hold. Meanwhile, what we eat actually plays a relatively minor role in health. Public-health researchers have found that when it comes to modifiable determinants of health (that is, the things over which we have some individual or societal control, as opposed to genetics, which we can't change), eating and physical activity combined account for only about *10 percent* of population health outcomes.[16] Other health-related behaviors account for only another 20 percent.

What's really insidious is that nutrition researchers and the health-and-wellness media—two groups of people who are, again, all too human—tend to play off each other in a way that further reinforces diet culture. You might think that to get a job reporting about nutrition you need to have at least some background in science. Not so: science journalists of all kinds usually go into their chosen beat without any scientific training. Instead they learn on the job, as most of my colleagues and I did when we started reporting on nutrition and other "wellness" topics. (As an undergraduate I majored in rhetoric and French literature, then went straight into my first nutrition-journalism jobs from there; not until years later did I attend graduate school to study nutrition and public health.) Unfortunately, that lack of training can make science seem a little opaque and mystical to reporters, who often treat both science and scientists as authorities and are therefore unlikely to dig deeply into research findings, let alone question them.[17]

Thus, what gets reported to the public is typically a watered-down version of the scientific findings in question, based not on the full text of the study but on the abstract or even just a *press release* about the findings. (It's a horrifying practice but also an understandable one, given how overworked and underpaid most journalists are; this isn't a problem with individual report-ers so much as it is with the practices of the media companies that employ them, and with the industry as a whole.) Scientists themselves often contribute to this dynamic by summarizing their own results in a simplified and sensationalized way, which helps them attract media attention that increases their visibility, thereby upping their ability to get funding for future research — and then the cycle continues. Again, this isn't the fault of the individual scientists, who are just trying to get by in a field that, like many others, rewards bombastic self-promotion and dis-courages quiet deliberation; this is an issue with the field itself. The book-publishing industry plays a role here, too, giving these scientists and journalists book deals that further spread their hyperbolic messages.

In the publish-or-perish climate that characterizes today's scientific-research community and the media and publishing industries, scientists and reporters are in a symbiotic relation-ship that helps feed both groups' need for a steady stream of information that sells. At this point in history, fearmongering messages about food and body size sell — that's simply the cul-ture we live in — so that's what we keep getting from scientific publications and the media that reports on them. Thus diet-culture beliefs about food and bodies get perpetuated under the guise of "the latest science," with no regard for the nuances of what the science really says (and doesn't say). So if you're a consumer of media about nutrition and health, keep in mind that the fields of nutrition science and health journalism—just like all corners of the health-and-wellness industry—are, with few exceptions, caught up in diet culture. Their findings should be taken with a *huge* grain of salt.

Other groups that have largely bought into diet culture include dietitians, "holistic" nutritionists, and other "wellness" professionals who focus on food, as well as doctors, nurses, and others in the medical field. Doctors, in fact, are the most frequent source of weight stigma reported by women and the second-most-frequent source reported by men. (The No. 1 source for men? Classmates in school settings.)[18] Research has found that both implicit and explicit anti-fat stigma is just as prevalent among medical doctors as it is in the general public.[19] Dietitians, meanwhile, have a greater prevalence of eating disorders and orthorexia than the overall population.[20] I recently witnessed a discussion among a bunch of dietitians that devolved into an unscientific laundry list of personal diet tips: "When I have [food X] in my house, it is very hard to eat just the few small [Xs] that it would take to not gain weight," and "I had a craving for [food A] and I knew it was just a sugar fix I was looking for, so I tried [diet food A] and [diet food B] mixed in [diet food C]." (A number of my clients have been given similar advice—again, based on personal experience rather than scientific evidence—by their doctors: "The X diet is the only one that ever worked for me.")

Health professionals aren't gods. They are human beings who received their training in a certain cultural context—and at this point in history, that context is fatphobic and food-phobic. That's worth keeping in mind whenever you talk with a health-care provider. They may have advanced degrees and valuable knowledge in many areas, but unless they've done the work to unlearn diet-culture beliefs, odds are their ideas about food, movement, and body size will be steeped in weight stigma and "good/bad" food rhetoric—which, as we've seen, can do a lot more harm than good to their clients' health.

Social Justice

When diet culture demonizes certain foods while elevating others, it conveniently distracts our attention from the real issues. Rather than admitting that its methods of deprivation, restriction, and self-blame don't work—and that they instead actively harm our physical and mental health—diet culture points the finger at particular foods it falsely labels as "toxic," "addictive," or just plain "bad." From cookies to gluten to tomatoes, the foods that diet culture demonizes vary based on trends and flimsy science. But for the vast majority of people, restricting those foods never leads to long-term benefits. That's because the problem isn't the food. The problem is the deprivation, shame, and guilt that diet culture instills in us, which leads us to swing wildly between restricting and feeling out of control, never able to access the peace and trust in our bodies that is our birthright. The problem is diet culture itself.

Ditching the "good" and "bad" labels, then, is key to dismantling diet culture as a larger system. Refusing to demonize or elevate foods means letting go of the racist, colonialist mind-set that holds certain foods and certain bodies as "better" than others. Ceasing to moralize about food also helps shift the focus back to the determinants of health—social inequality, poverty, chronic stress, discrimination—that matter a lot more than how much kale you eat.

In that sense, no longer labeling food as "good" or "bad" is essential to the project of social justice, of creating a society where people have equal access to *truly* holistic well-being. Sure, you can still fight to make fruits and vegetables more available in low-income communities, not because "processed" foods are "bad" or because there's a supposed "obesity epidemic," but because all people deserve access to all kinds of food. The more important issue, though, is making the more-significant determinants of health—freedom from oppression, a sense of financial security, a safe place to live, and *enough* food on the table consistently—accessible to everyone, no matter their background or body size. Once we all stop obsessing over what we eat, we'll be a lot more capable of collectively addressing those issues.

CHAPTER 10

Health at Every Size — and Body Liberation

Given that diet culture's version of "health" is so damaging to people's well-being, it's tempting to throw up your hands and say "Fuck it" on matters of health. And I'm here to tell you that's a valid response. Sure, I'm a health professional, but health is *not* a moral obligation: you aren't required to pursue it in order to prove your worthiness. In fact, if you've been traumatized by the pursuit of health in the past, as so many of us have been, you might need some time off to heal—and that's perfectly OK. It doesn't mean anything bad about you as a person, no matter what diet culture may have led you to believe. As health coach Ragen Chastain says, "Running a marathon and having a Net-flix marathon are morally equivalent activities." Plus, people aren't always able to pursue or prioritize their health because of circumstances such as poverty, food and job insecurity, caregiving duties, disabilities, or a host of other reasons.

Your health isn't entirely within your control, either, despite what diet culture wants you to think. Health isn't something you can wrestle into submission by sheer force; certain circumstances beyond our control—genetics, socioeconomic status, experiences of stigma, environmental exposures—can affect our health outcomes. We can't permanently change our body size through food intake and exercise, the way we've been told we can, and the same is true of our health—which, of course, is *not* dependent on body size. That is, even if everyone ate the exact same things and moved their bodies in the exact same ways, we'd all still have different health outcomes because of genetic differences, experiences of poverty and discrimination, and even deprivation that our mothers experienced during pregnancy. Many things contribute to health, meaning it's not all down to personal responsibility, the way diet culture wants us to believe—not by a long shot.

If and when you are ready to think about matters of health, an alternative exists to diet culture's way of doing things. It's called Health At Every Size® (aka HAES®, trademarked by its founders to keep it from getting co-opted by diet culture), and it's a weight-inclusive, anti-diet approach to health care that's designed to help you take care of your body without trying to shrink it. HAES was formally developed in the 1990s, in response to all of the existing and emerging research showing that intentional weight loss doesn't work and causes more harm than good, as well as the growing evidence of weight stigma in society and medicine. Born of a union between the fat-liberation movement and a group of dietitians and therapists sympathetic to their cause, HAES is a method that health-care providers can use to help support the well-being of people in larger bodies without falling into the trap of recommending weight loss.

The principles of the HAES paradigm are diametrically opposed to those of diet culture. Those principles are:

- providing weight-inclusive care that accepts and respects body diversity and refuses to demonize certain weights or elevate others;
- supporting health-related policies and practices that help people's well-being in a *truly* holistic sense, including their physical, emotional, social, spiritual, and economic needs;
- refusing to blame people for their health outcomes;

- acknowledging the biases that health-care providers hold, and working to end discrimination and stigma based on body size or any other form of identity;
- providing respectful care that acknowledges the intersecting identities people hold (among them race, gender, and socioeconomic status) and the ways those identities can interact with weight stigma;
- promoting intuitive eating and a pleasurable relationship with food, rather than external "eating plans" designed to shrink the body; and
- supporting a joyful relationship with movement that allows people of all sizes, shapes, and abilities to determine their own level of engagement in physical activity.[1]

HAES provides an answer to the question, "If I'm going to step outside diet culture, what should I do to take care of my health?" Not only does HAES focus on *behaviors* you can adopt to help your health (because weight is not a behavior), it helps reduce the toll of weight stigma on people who live in larger bodies. In that sense, it plays an important role in supporting people's health. HAES also embraces the natural size diversity that exists in the world. Whereas some critics argue that HAES and the anti-diet movement in general "promote obesity," the reality is that this paradigm promotes people in *all* body sizes taking care of themselves to the best of their abilities and living free of stigma and discrimination. HAES helps people of all shapes and sizes to feel at peace with their bodies, the way we all deserve to feel — no matter what diet culture claims.

A HAES approach acknowledges that health looks different for everyone, and that numerous factors go into our overall health that have nothing to do with the size of our body or the food we eat or the amount of exercise we get. The HAES paradigm recognizes that true well-being includes social connections, meaningful

work, fulfillment in our lives, and a sense of purpose. It empha-
sizes that all aspects of our lives be cared for. And rather than forcing ourselves to shrink our bodies, it fosters self-compassion.

Self-Care, Not Self-Control

One of my favorite mantras for describing a HAES approach to
health is "self-care, not self-control." It's what a peaceful, intuitive relationship with food and your body is all about. When it
comes to the food part, an approach based on self-care rather
than self-control goes something like this:

- making food choices that care for your mental health—
  honoring desire, satisfaction, spontaneity, and flexibility—
  as well as your physical health;
- pursuing joy and pleasure in food rather than deprivation
  and restriction;
- caring for your body by meeting its need for food—enough
  food overall, and a wide variety of foods that bring you both
  energy and happiness (and that definitely includes dessert,
  by the way);
- grabbing a bite or a drink with friends after work without
  worrying about what you ate earlier in the day;
- serving yourself enough to truly satisfy your hunger, which
  might mean going back for seconds;
- packing snacks when you know you're going to be out for a
  while; and
- having, say, hot chocolate on a cold day because it's comforting, or watermelon on a hot day because it's refreshing.

Diet culture messes with our ability to engage in these acts
of self-care by putting the focus on control. It's constantly telling

us that we "shouldn't" need or want as much food as we do, "shouldn't" be as hungry as we are. It tells us to control our desires, to fight our body's natural cues. It keeps us stuck in mere survival mode, obsessing over food and our bodies, at the expense of so many other things we could be doing with our time and energy.

But guess what? We don't need to impose famine on ourselves. You can take care of your body's needs so that you feel safe. And that leaves you free to work on building the life you always wanted — one that supports your personal relationships, professional goals, intellectual passions, creative pursuits, and so much more.

"Self-care, not self-control" likewise means letting your weight settle where it may. As my fellow HAES dietitian Dana Sturtevant succinctly puts it, "It's not possible to heal our relationship with food and body while trying to control the size and shape of our body." In other words, you *have* to let that shit go if you want to stop feeling unhinged around food. Diet culture makes this difficult, but getting to a place where you're not actively trying to shrink your body is an essential ingredient in your physical and mental well-being. Breaking free from diet culture means breaking free from *all* of it, including idealizing smaller bodies and equating thinness with health and moral virtue. In a truly self-caring relationship with your body, weight loss or management can never be the goal.

How exactly does that work, in terms of health? The thing is, your body is *way* smarter than you think. It will determine whatever weight it needs to be when you're practicing self-care behaviors to the best of your abilities, to the extent that you're able to prioritize self-care. Your body will figure it out. Remember the weight set range from Chapter 3? When you stop trying to control your size, your body will eventually find that set range and stay there. When you're consistently practicing self-care and you haven't engaged in dieting or disordered-eating behaviors for a good long time (like months or years), it's likely that whatever size you are is the size your body wants to be.

I always tell my clients that saying you want to be a certain size or weight is putting the cart before the horse. The horse is your genetics, your history, your socioeconomic status, and many other things outside your control, as well as your behaviors, which include your relationship with food—not just *what* you eat but *how* you eat. Like the horse pulling the cart, letting go of dieting behaviors and starting to nourish yourself in an intuitive way pulls your weight along to wherever it wants to be. *Your body is not meant to be at a weight that it can sustain only through restriction.*

Your weight may increase as a result of letting go of restriction and deprivation, or it may decrease because your body is no longer in starvation mode and holding on for dear life. Or your weight may stay the same, plus or minus some fluctuations as your body adjusts to having its needs met. Once you're in the habit of nourishing yourself consistently, honoring your hunger, and not restricting or avoiding any foods (other than for legitimate medical reasons), your weight will find its set range and stay there (barring things like pregnancy or medication changes). We can't predict what's going to happen to your weight when you give up dieting, but it doesn't matter one bit in terms of your health or your worthiness.

Taking the Focus off Weight

In Chapter 5 we discussed what to do if your weight is making you *physically uncomfortable* in your body. We talked about exploring the role diet culture and weight stigma play in creating that discomfort, which includes asking yourself some hard questions: What are those feelings of discomfort really about? Are they because certain things are harder to do—and if so, what are those things? Then, instead of trying to shrink your body in order to be able to do what you want to do, you can work on weight-inclusive ways of getting there.

You might want to walk up a flight of stairs without getting winded, for example. Augmenting your capacity to accomplish that does *not* require shrinking yourself. That capacity is actually a function of building strength and stamina for that particular activity, which has nothing to do with your size. Even if you have a disability that prevents you from walking, you can increase your mobility in ways that don't involve intentional weight loss. "The pillars of athletics are strength, stamina, flexibility, and sport-specific technique," says health coach Ragen Chastain. "So if somebody is worried about mobility I would suggest they look at strength, stamina, and flexibility, then look at ways to improve those things and see what happens, rather than trying to manipulate body size." As the holder of the Guinness World Record for heaviest woman ever to complete a marathon, Chastain knows that building those athletic capacities "is something that works at all sizes, whereas weight loss is something that works for almost no one."

That's the thing: as I've underlined throughout this book, trying to shrink your body is not merely ineffective in the long run but *actively causes harm.* And that's true for people in bodies of all sizes—including the very largest ones—and of all shapes and abilities. In this fat-stigmatizing society, it's likely you'll feel discomfort at a higher weight that is not directly *caused* by that weight. Of course, it's also difficult to move through the world when you're living in a body labeled "too big" for things such as theater seats and doctors' blood-pressure cuffs. But once again, *your body is not the problem.* Diet culture is the problem.

Awakening to this cultural bias is imperative for you as an individual and for society as a whole. Once we understand that diet culture is an oppressive system robbing us of our human rights, we can start healing from it at the individual level—and start tearing it down at the collective level. In the most basic sense, when we stop feeling bad about our bodies, we'll stop forking over our time, money, well-being, and happiness to diet culture. So remember that you need not shrink your body for *anyone*—not even "for yourself," as today's sneaky diet ads urge. (Would you have the desire to shrink your body in the first place if it weren't for this toxic culture?) And even if you're swayed by messages to go on a diet, your body has a mind of its own: it's not going to obey your diet culture–driven demands (at least not for long, and not without doing significant damage to your mental health and your relationship with food).

There's no magic diet. For the vast majority of people, there's no way to lose weight and keep it off for more than a handful of years. Even if you're one of the minuscule percentage of people for whom that does seem to be happening, there's still no diet that won't create chaos in your relationship with food. There's no form of intentional weight loss that lets you live peacefully with food and your body. As one of my podcast listeners revealed in an iTunes review, "I'm in the 5% of people who have lost a significant amount of weight and have stayed there for 5 years. But guess what: I found this podcast after searching for 'binge eating' in the search bar here. Yeah. Exactly."

So let's stop believing diet culture's false promises—and recognize that there's no way to play by its rules and win. You don't have to keep chasing that dragon. It's a quest that can end only in misery, and meanwhile there's so much life happening right here, right now. Instead of devoting your time on this planet to finding the perfect diet, work to make peace with food and your body so that you can free your mind for the things that truly matter in life.

You might start by throwing away your scale—or smashing it, as many of my clients and colleagues have done. The bathroom scale is a tool of diet culture, and therefore an instrument of oppression. Keeping a scale in your home doesn't provide any benefits, and it only hurts your self-worth to attach your feelings about yourself to an arbitrary number that means nothing about you as a person. Scales mire you in the diet mentality, focusing on your weight and consciously or unconsciously trying to change it. Think about all the times you've had your day ruined the moment you stepped on that hunk of metal and plastic. Has the scale *ever* provided any long-lasting sense of self-acceptance or peace? Or has it simply kept you coming back for more — and feeling that whatever number you saw was never "good enough?" If you've struggled with the scale, now is a great time to get rid of it. Remind yourself you're much more than a number, then chuck that thing on the trash pile.

Oh, and buy bigger clothes. Your body will thank you every moment of the day.

Out with Exercise, In with Movement

"The truth is, we don't need as much exercise as we think we do," says Jessi Haggerty, a personal trainer and registered dietitian with a private practice in Somerville, Massachusetts, who uses a HAES approach in her work. "There's such an emphasis on high-intensity exercise and getting so many hours of exercise every week, and I'm always like, 'We don't need to do that much. And it doesn't have to all be structured.' " Despite the "somewhat superficial" reasons that drove her to become a personal trainer — and the diet culture–infused training she went through to get her certification — Haggerty ultimately found that the most effective and rewarding approach is to take weight loss out of the equation; instead she focuses on helping her clients *be present* in their bodies during physical activity. She also recommends stepping away from fitness trackers, which interfere with that ability to be present. "Delete MyFitnessPal," she says. "Take off your FitBit."

Years ago Haggerty had her own struggles with food and her body, which forced her to reckon with her relationship to exercise. "I think a good question to always ask is, 'Why am I doing this right now?' and being really honest with yourself," she says. "When I started asking myself that question, the amount of exercise I was doing decreased significantly. Because I was like, 'Either I don't have a good reason, or I can't think of a reason unrelated to manipulating my body in some way.'" For Haggerty, cutting back on physical activity was instrumental in healing her relationship with her body. It was also hard, because so much of her identity—both as a personal trainer and as a person—was wrapped up in how much she exercised. "It's a weird thing to say, 'Oh yeah, I'm a personal trainer but I don't go to the gym,'" she says.

In fact, most gyms are hotbeds of diet culture, and many people would do well to step away from them—and perhaps from the concept of "exercise" entirely. That word was originally used to describe both military drills and driving livestock to the field to plow, so it's no surprise that people view it in a punishing way (or that certain fitness classes bill themselves as "boot camps"). In diet culture, exercise is treated as a body-shrinking tool, just like dieting or "watching what you eat." For many of us, it brings back memories of high-school gym class and being picked last for dodgeball. It's about "working out," "no pain, no gain," instructors yelling at you, and being ashamed that you can't keep up. It's no fun.

Movement, on the other hand, is free of the connotations of a military boot camp. It doesn't have to look a certain way or burn a certain number of calories or get your heart rate up to a certain level. It just is what it is, and it includes everything from walking to the mailbox to paddling around in a lake to weeding the garden to helping your sister redecorate. It can be structured or unstructured. It can be joyful, like going to a dance party (or having a spontaneous one in your living room);

competitive, like playing a game of basketball or challenging a friend to a race; or utilitarian, like carrying groceries from the store to your apartment a few blocks away. It can be done to help your mental health, like going to a yoga class or taking a walk to clear your head. It can also be done to help you feel more comfortable in your body, like physical therapy to heal an injury or manage chronic pain, but its purpose isn't to shrink or reshape your body. Movement is intuitive, flexible, and unrelated to diet culture. So I'd encourage you to stop exercising and start just *moving* in whatever way feels good to you, without any expectations of what it's "supposed" to look like.

Of course, if you're struggling with an eating disorder or an exercise compulsion, the amount of movement your body needs might be *zero* right now — because it needs to heal, and because you need to heal your relationship with it. Trust that instinct, and give yourself time to recover. Eventually you'll be able to come back to movement in a way that's free from diet culture's intrusions.

You may have always thought of yourself as someone who avoids exercise, but that's merely the flip side of the compulsive-exercise coin. In both cases, the conversation about movement has been dominated by control and guilt and *should*s and all this other diet-culture bullshit — not exactly conducive to feeling joy about movement. Whether you're following diet culture's rules because you think you should, or you're rebelling against those rules by not moving much at all, you don't have any *internal* motivation to move your body. There's no intrinsic desire to do it.

Both compulsive exercisers and movement-averse folks therefore need permission *not* to move in any structured way — unless and until they genuinely want to do so. Remember that movement, just like every other aspect of health, is *not* a moral obligation. What would it feel like if you had total license not to engage in any form of movement unless you genuinely wanted to (or unless it was a built-in part of your day, like walking home with those groceries)? What would it feel like to kick the diet-culture drill sergeant out of your head? You might focus exclusively on detecting the subtle signs that your body craves movement or rest, and practice responding to those in ways that are easy, low-key, and fun. The more you can practice noticing and responding to those small desires for movement, the more you'll cultivate the joyful aspect of movement and the less you'll heed the drill-sergeant voice. Eventually you'll find a way of relating to movement that neither follows diet-culture rules nor rebels against them.

For transgender folks, I know that exercising to try to reduce gender dysphoria is a common practice. I'm not here to condemn anyone's efforts to align with their true gender—I support your doing what you need to do to feel less dysphoric and take care of your mental health, and as a cisgender woman I can't even pretend to know what dysphoria feels like. But what I do know—and what I hope you'll consider—is that beauty standards for *all* genders are entangled in diet culture. As nonbinary trans psychologist Sand Chang pointed out in Chapter 1, those standards don't leave room for people of *any* gender who fall outside its oppressive body-size and body-shape norms. So even if you're engaging in dieting and exercise to address gender dysphoria, I invite you to consider the role that diet culture plays in your relationship with food, movement, and your body, and see if there's a way to break free from its hold on you. (For more on these ideas, check out *Food Psych* with Sand at christyharrison .com/150, or my talk with trans writer and activist Caleb Luna at christyharrison.com/142.)

Dealing with Doctors

Another important step to take toward Health At Every Size is finding health-care professionals who will actively support your health, not add to your internalized weight stigma. If you have a doctor who persists in holding on to diet-culture beliefs about weight—even after you've tried setting boundaries with that provider—you have every right to fire them and find a new doctor. Remember, doctors work for *you*, not the other way around. A doctor is a service provider, just like a plumber or a car mechanic or a hairstylist. If you didn't like the way someone cut your hair, would you go back to them, or would you seek out a new stylist? If your mechanic constantly shamed you about, say, the color of your car, wouldn't you consider finding a new mechanic? The same approach should apply to medical providers: You don't have to settle for health-care services that make you feel crappy and ashamed. From doctors and nurses to therapists and personal trainers, you deserve to find health professionals who will listen to you and provide evidence-based care. And there *are* providers out there who get it—it just may take a little work to find them. (Check out the Resources section at the back of the book for some recommendations on how to do that.)

Even if your provider is not familiar with HAES, you can give them a crash course in its principles and ask them to treat you using the following guidelines (I developed these through the process of counseling hundreds of people in my private practice and online courses):

Guidelines for Health-Care Providers to Prevent Weight Stigma and Disordered Eating

- Focus on evidence-based interventions to improve health, which do *not* include weight loss. Don't use body mass index (BMI) as a measure of health; using this measure is likely to lead to misdiagnosis for both larger- and smaller-bodied people.[2]

- Recommend the same evidence-based interventions to patients in larger bodies as you would to patients in smaller bodies. For example, if someone in a larger body has a bacterial infection, prescribe antibiotics. If they have knee pain, recommend physical therapy. Don't recommend weight loss.

- Don't require patients to step on the scale, except in cases of true medical necessity such as administering anesthesia or monitoring their recovery from a restrictive-eating disorder. In those cases, allow patients to stand backward on the scale without looking, and don't show or tell them the number (or let anyone on your staff do so), including on visit-summary printouts.

- Don't give nutrition recommendations to anyone with a history of chronic dieting or other forms of disordered eating, except perhaps in cases where the scientific-evidence base for the recommendation is airtight (for example, celiac disease or anaphylactic allergy). For conditions where the scientific evidence for food restrictions is inconclusive, nonexistent, or emerging—such as irritable bowel syndrome, thyroid disease, or Crohn's disease—limit your recommendations to non-nutritional interventions. Always refer patients to dietitians and psychotherapists experienced in the treatment of disordered eating.

- Don't recommend exercise as an intervention unless you have a deep understanding of a patient's relationship with physical activity. Many people are at risk for compulsive exercise, particularly those with a history of dieting and other forms of disordered eating. It's also extremely common for people to have traumatic histories with physical activity that lead them to avoid it. When in doubt, don't prescribe movement.

- Equip your facility with size-inclusive blood-pressure cuffs, exam tables, gowns, and other equipment, as well as high-capacity, arm-free chairs and spaces for wheelchairs and other mobility aids.
- Keep weight-stigmatizing or food-shaming television programming, health and fitness magazines, and diet books out of your waiting area.

HAES and Eating-Disorder Recovery

From 2014 to 2015, alongside my private practice, I worked part-time for an organization that offers meal support to clients recovering from eating disorders. Meal support is a wonderfully weird cross between outpatient nutrition counseling, psychotherapy, and friendship that involves helping clients order food according to their recovery meal plans, manage any freak-outs about the food, and have as pleasant a time as possible while eating. That job is where I first met Sushi Pizza. That's not her real name, of course, but one time we went out to a restaurant that served, among other things, pizza topped with sashimi and nori, and when I told the guy I was seeing (now my husband) about the meal I'd had with my client, he gave her that nickname as a way to mention a client without breaking anonymity. (Never mind that *I* was actually the one who'd ordered the pizza.)

Like many people with eating disorders, Sushi Pizza had a major fear of pizza. She wouldn't touch the piece I offered her that night, and it generally took some coaxing to get her to eat the (non-pizza) carbs at our dinners two or three times a week. This was a woman who'd struggled with restrictive anorexia for more than half her life, who saw herself as fat despite being emaciated, and who'd been in and out of more treatment programs than I could keep track of. In many ways, she was diet culture's quintessential picture of someone with an eating disorder. And although eating disorders can present themselves in a million other ways and most often *don't* result in emaciation or stints in treatment centers, diet culture's skewed views mean that people like Sushi Pizza are more likely to get recognized and get help, whereas others do not.

You might think this combination of anorexia and privilege would make Sushi Pizza unsympathetic to the plight of larger-bodied folks or resistant to a HAES approach, but you'd be wrong. One day, some time after she'd started working with me in private practice in addition to the meal support, she sat in my office sharing how she'd fallen short on some of her attempts at breaking free from the eating disorder that week. I was empathizing with how difficult it was to recover in this culture where disordered eating is normalized, and something inspired me to blurt out, "Take a look at the chair you're sitting on right now— have you ever wondered why it has no arms?" Her eyes widened as she considered what I was saying, not quite understanding yet. "Not everyone can fit into chairs with arms," I continued, "just like not everyone can fit into airplane seats or booths at restaurants. A lot of public spaces in our world aren't made to accommodate people in larger bodies, so it's unfortunately a privilege to be able to fit into those spaces—a privilege that you and I both have, but that many of my clients don't. And I want my office to be inclusive of everyone. Hence, no arms on the chairs."

In that moment, I saw something click for Sushi Pizza. For the rest of that session, she reflected on the injustices of the world for people in larger bodies, and I introduced her to some of the basic principles of HAES: that weight doesn't equal health, that restrictive and disordered eating cause harm for people of *all* sizes, and that weight stigma is a form of discrimination just like racism, sexism, or homophobia. As someone already sensitive to social-justice issues, she readily grasped the idea that social justice extends to body size; of *course* it does.

That conversation lit a fire for her, and over the coming weeks and months she began to deepen her understanding of HAES and justice for all bodies. Despite all her eating-disorder treatments, she had never heard these concepts before; now she was talking about them with everyone she knew. "I will forever be grateful for you introducing me to the importance of Health At Every Size," she wrote to me recently. "HAES was a final call to action I didn't know I needed. Developing a deeper under-standing of its principles helped me begin to direct my anger away from my body and myself, and instead aim it toward the systems that perpetuate diet culture and the hyper-fixation on a particular body size. It's a guiding light that consistently redirects me toward the path of recovery when I stumble or stray."

In many corners of the eating-disorder-treatment world, a HAES approach is considered essential for helping people recover. Our culture's disordered relationship with food and bodies is a major factor in the development of eating disorders, the thinking goes; if we want to prevent and heal these disor-ders, we have to offer a space free from diet culture and the pressure to lose weight. We need another way.

Every major eating-disorder conference I've been to has had at least a few sessions that advocate the HAES approach and discuss why it's a best practice for treating eating disorders.[3] Dozens of my colleagues in the eating-disorder field have been professionally and personally affected by HAES. Among them are psychothera-pist Lisa DuBreuil, whom the paradigm endowed with a deep com-passion and appreciation for her own larger body—and an understanding of how to care for it in a way that wasn't infused with diet culture. "Health At Every Size really brought me over the finish line, so to speak, in my eating disorder recovery," says DuBreuil. She first learned about HAES at an eating-disorder conference when she was just starting to specialize in this field; now, some twenty years later, DuBreuil is one of the leading eating-disorder-treatment providers who practice from a HAES perspective.

Unfortunately, some darker corners of the eating-disorder-treatment world are still very much a part of diet culture. These recesses tend to have the most corporate influence: big, national companies with treatment centers across the country that offer an "obesity" track alongside traditional eating-disorder-recovery tracks such as binge eating and anorexia. In such settings, weight loss is often encouraged as part of the recovery process. Outpatient dietitians, doctors, and psychotherapists who work with eating disorders in private practice often buy into the diet-culture hype, too, because they're human — and that sadly often translates to them undermining their clients' recovery.

In coordinating care for my clients with eating disorders, I've heard fellow health-care providers say things like "Well, if she really weren't bingeing anymore, she should be losing weight," and "Try to encourage him to cut back on calorie-dense foods." Remember: there's zero evidence that *any* weight-loss strategy works in the long run for more than a tiny percentage of people, or that people inevitably lose weight when they stop bingeing. Instead there's abundant evidence that pushing intentional weight loss and shaming people for their weight result in worse health outcomes, *including higher rates of disordered eating.* Of all people, health-care providers who specialize in the treatment of eating disorders should know this. But too many of them don't. So if you're looking for a provider to help you recover from an eating disorder, do your homework and make sure they're versed in HAES — either by asking them during your initial consultation, or by looking in specialized HAES directories (such as the Resources section at the back of the book) for referrals.

Some eating-disorder-treatment providers may shy away from HAES because of a misconception that it means people are automatically "healthy at any size," including at starved weights. But that's not what HAES is about at all. It doesn't mean that you're automatically healthy whatever size you're at right now, but rather — in the case of eating disorders — that it's not your weight that matters, it's the presence or absence of disordered behaviors. For people who are in weight-suppressed bodies due to eating disorders, the real driver of the problem is the behaviors—the restriction, the bulimia, the drug abuse, the compulsive exercise, or whatever else people are doing to try to lose weight. So recovery isn't a simple matter of making emaciated people gain weight and assuming everything will be fine, or assuming that people are fine because they're *not* emaciated. Instead, it's about getting to the bottom of the disordered behaviors, then removing those behaviors and allowing the body to restore itself to a weight at which the medical complications and the disordered thoughts subside. Once again, weight is just a side effect—the cart getting pulled along behind the horse. When it comes to disordered eating, the real issue is the behaviors. So don't go around thinking *It's OK that I'm "underweight" because of Health At Every Size* when in fact you're super disordered with food and it's jeopardizing your health. When you have an eating disorder, you're *not* fine, no matter your size. You might call eating disorders "Un-health At Every Size."

As the antidote to disordered eating, HAES is an essential tool for eating-disorder recovery. Anyone with disordered eating needs to know that no matter what weight they end up at, they'll be OK—that higher weights don't automatically equal poor health. People of *all* sizes can benefit from HAES principles. That includes the millions of people whom diet culture might deem "not thin enough" to have an eating disorder—like many of the people you've heard from in this book—as well as people who fit the stereotypical profile, such as Sushi Pizza.

Speaking of whom: Sushi Pizza is not yet fully recovered, but she's more committed to recovery than ever before. Rather than bouncing in and out of intensive treatment centers, she is finally living the life that had always felt out of reach. She even occasionally eats pizza, and she loves her nickname—in fact, she asked that I use it when telling her story here.

Reframing Our Relationship with the Body

Health At Every Size is a powerful tool for health care. Even more important, however, is the right to live peacefully in your body whether or not you pursue health *at all*—which, remember, no one is under any obligation to do. Diet culture is a system of oppression, and in order to combat any such system we need a new way of relating to one another and to ourselves. It's not enough to know what we *don't* want in our lives, although that's a huge part of the battle. We also need a framework for understanding and pursuing what we *do* want. In the case of building a system beyond diet culture, it means we need a new way of relating to bodies in general—ours and everyone else's. We need a philosophy that promotes being at peace with the body.

This idea of *body peace* goes by many different names and comes in many different flavors: body positivity, body love, body confidence, body neutrality. One of my favorites is the term *body respect* (also the title of a great book by my colleagues Lindo Bacon and Lucy Aphramor[4]), because while it's hard to jump to accepting your body or even loving your body when you're at war with it, it *is* possible to show it some respect—to stop denigrating it, to stop starving and punishing it, and to start caring for it. I also like the concept of *body trust* (developed by dietitian Dana Sturtevant and mental-health counselor Hilary Kinavey through their company, Be Nourished[5]), because learning to trust your body in matters of food and movement is essential. Getting back to your intuition about food—an inner wisdom we were all born with—is a matter of trust, and it's an entirely different paradigm than having diet culture constantly sowing self-doubt in your mind. As we've seen, your body must relearn to trust *you*, too—to trust that you're not going to put it through another famine, that you're not going to expose it to deprivation again—in order to relax and allow you to stop feeling out of control around food.

The idea of *body appreciation* is great, too, and it's been helpful to me in my own recovery from diet culture. Even if I'm having a day where I'm not jazzed about what my body looks like, I can still appreciate it for everything it *does*. Lungs breathing, heart beating, cells regenerating, neurons firing, digestive system digesting—all of these things happen without my conscious control, allowing me to be here on this planet experiencing life. Without my body, I would cease to exist in this form, in this world. Like a reliable old car, my body gets me where I want to go. As much as I might sometimes wish it looked more put-together and worry about how people might be judging it, I'm grateful to it for allowing me to be here and move through life. Trying to have gratitude for those basic gifts of existence can take the focus (and the onus) off the way particular body parts look—and whether or not they "measure up" to the impossible standards set by diet culture.

Likewise helpful, if a bit trickier, is the notion of *body acceptance*. On one hand, it's incredibly important to accept the size of your body and stop trying to shrink it, because to the extent that you don't accept it, diet culture still has a hold on you. On the other hand, some people in marginalized bodies— particularly trans and nonbinary folks—may find it extremely hard, even offensive, to think about accepting their bodies exactly as they are. Body acceptance is a fraught concept that way. If you're struggling with gender dysphoria, gender-affirming surgery can literally be a lifesaving procedure, given that dysphoria contributes to the disproportionately high rates of suicide among trans folks. As psychologist Sand Chang explains, body acceptance for a trans person might mean accepting yourself *as* transgender, accepting that your gender identity doesn't match with your sex assigned at birth, and accepting that you need medical intervention to come into alignment with your true gender identity. Accepting your body exactly as is might not be an option in those cases—and that's OK.

Ultimately, the term I like best for describing how to relate to the body without the influence of diet culture is *body liberation:* to me it's sort of what all the other terms are getting at, in their own ways. I first heard it from writer and activist Jes Baker, and I like it because it spotlights the idea of freedom from stigma and oppression for *all* bodies. Body liberation is inextricable from social justice. It encompasses people of all sizes, races, ethnicities, abilities and disabilities, gender identities, sexual orientations, ages, and all the rest. It *has* to include all of those facets of our identities, because they intersect in our bodies and are inseparable from one another. None of us is moving through the world with a single identity. "If I can't be positive in my blackness, and I can't be positive in my queerness, and I can't be positive in my neuro-divergence, then it doesn't matter if I'm totally OK being a size [X]," activist and author Sonya Renee Taylor says. This is why I find *body liberation* the best term to describe what we're striving for.

This is a systemic issue—one that goes far beyond individual empowerment. It's crucial for people to make peace with themselves and feel comfortable in their own skin, but the work doesn't end there. Individuals wouldn't need to undertake these self-empowerment journeys of learning to love and accept their bodies if systemic forms of oppression didn't cause people to believe their bodies are unacceptable. We wouldn't need a trademarked approach called Health At Every Size® if every health professional practiced that approach. And I could've written a totally different book—and followed a totally different career trajectory—if diet culture hadn't been so present in my life.

The fact that so many individuals are working to help so many others recover from diet culture underscores our need to address the root causes. As Archbishop Desmond Tutu said, "There comes a point where we need to stop just pulling people out of the river. We need to go upstream and find out why they're falling in."

We know, more or less, why people are falling into the river of diet culture, so now we need to make it stop. We need a movement for collective liberation and acceptance of all bodies — because that will eventually translate into self-acceptance for individuals. We need community-level and culture-wide changes.

I've said it before, and I'll say it again: we need to burn diet culture to the ground.

CHAPTER 11

The Power of Community

I've lived in New York City for fifteen years now, and what they say is true: most of the time you're bombarded with noise and stimulation and people crowding your personal space, because there are 8.6 million of us squished into a landmass that feels like the size of a shopping mall. If you don't want to have a total meltdown, you have to find ways to escape. My favorite is to go on a day trip to one of the local beaches, because for the same price as your commute to work, you can take the subway to a place that's worlds away from the daily grind. There's almost nothing I love more than seeing the towering chaos of the city fade into a distant speck across the sparkling water of Jamaica Bay, and trading in the concrete and sweat of a regular summer day in Brooklyn for sand and saltwater. (And of course it helps that I'm far enough into my diet-culture recovery that wearing a bathing suit in public no longer causes me to fold in on myself with anxiety.)

So one sweltering-hot summer Sunday seven or eight years ago, my sister and I hopped on the A train and headed down to Rockaway Beach. It was exactly the escape we needed. We lay on our towels and read, swam out over the roiling waves and floated in the calm waters beyond, and ate some kick-ass beachside tacos and ice cream. We stared out at the horizon and felt that deep, satisfying exhaustion that only a long day in the sun can bring.

By the time we swiped our MetroCards to head home, I felt completely relaxed and restored—as if I'd spent the day at a spa, for a fraction of the cost.

And then, suddenly, all those good feelings got ripped away. At the last subway stop on the sparkling bay, a man burst through the doors and started shouting obscenities and murderous threats as he stomped up and down the aisle, pausing to leer and shake his fist at frightened passengers along the way. "I'm gonna kill you," he yelled over and over, pacing wildly as the subway lurched and leaned. In an instant, it felt like every one of those relaxed, beachy vibes left my body. I'd seen my share of weird shit on the subway at that point, but nothing as overtly scary as this. I glanced around to see if anyone seemed like they were going to get up and try to calm this guy down or alert the conductor, but all I saw were panicked, pleading eyes. Everyone looked just as eager to get the hell out of there as I was.

At the next stop, my sister and I—along with a dozen or so other passengers—rushed through the doors of the now-nearly-empty subway car, where the man was still ranting and pacing, and huddled on the platform to await the next train. "Welcome back to the city," said someone else who'd clearly just come from the beach. We all laughed nervously, hearts still pounding, coming together in a moment of solidarity. "Seriously, that was terrifying," I said. My sister and I chatted with our fellow passengers for a few more minutes until the next train came, then we all went our separate ways.

Being trapped in a speeding metal tube with a stranger threatening to kill you is a situation I hope you never find yourself in. But—and this may seem like a stretch, so hear me out—in many ways my experience that day coming home from the beach is not dissimilar to the experience of being thrown back into diet culture when you're trying to escape it. You can read this book and immerse yourself in other anti-diet resources, which is awesome and *so* needed—like escaping from the harsh city to the rejuvenating beach—but you never know when someone with their own diet-y issues is going to burst into your subway car and stomp all over your vibe. And it's not their fault, either; they need anti-diet resources of their own but don't have access to them, just as too many people lack access to social services that could help them manage the mental illnesses or substance-use disorders that make them threaten strangers on trains.

In both cases, what people really need is *support*. They need communities to rally around them and help them heal the pain and trauma that are causing them to act out. When you're the person on the receiving end of someone's pro-diet-culture rant, meanwhile, getting support from others—and eventually, perhaps, offering support to those who need it—is essential for helping you weather that storm and stay on the anti-diet path. You need to develop a community that helps you hold on to your self-compassionate values in the midst of diet culture. You need people to vent to and commiserate with, to process the shock and trauma of living in a fatphobic society. You need people who can see the Life Thief for what it is, name the problem, and help you bounce back from the inevitable onslaught of body-negative, food-shaming messages that you're bound to receive in this culture. Because while recovering from diet culture is healing and rewarding in the long run, it's also swimming upstream in a culture that sees things so differently. We need to find communities to support and sustain us, so that doing the work to unlearn diet culture's rules and restrictions doesn't feel like we're out there all alone in the wilderness (or in a terrifying subway car).

"I think one of the hardest things is that we live in a world where literally everyone around you is constantly supporting and reinforcing your belief that it's functional and beneficial to try to control your weight, and that if you're not dieting there's something wrong with you," says health coach Isabel Foxen Duke, who specializes in helping people break free from diet culture. "And so being able to have a different opinion is really, really hard. I think there's no way of making that un-hard—which is why developing a body-positive community, whether that be on the internet or anywhere else, is so important." Even changing your social-media feeds and subscribing to anti-diet podcasts is a way to help create a community for yourself that supports your recovery. "Surrounding yourself with body-positive culture is such a big part of the game, because our ability to perceive things as negative or positive is so heavily affected by culture," Duke explains.

To change how we perceive our bodies, we must put ourselves in a cultural milieu that portrays *all* bodies in a positive way. We have to create a little bubble around ourselves to help us push back against the entrenched diet-culture messages that we'll inevitably get from friends, family, medical providers, and the world at large. There's such a daily barrage of those messages that it's crucial to have a place in which we can be safe and process all that noise. If we want an alternative to diet culture, we have to actively seek out and create *anti-diet* culture for ourselves.

Diet culture, by the way, uses community support to its advantage *all the time.* Ever since the mid-twentieth century, when TOPS and Overeaters Anonymous and Weight Watchers started hosting their weight-loss support groups, diet culture has harnessed the power of community to make its messages stick (even if it could never bring about sustainable weight loss for more than a minuscule percentage of people). So if we're going to fight the Life Thief and take back all the things it stole from us, we need to reclaim our right to community support, too. And the first step in that process is realizing we're not alone in having struggled under the oppression of diet culture.

It's Not Just You

For much of her life, Rebekah Taussig, now a disability-rights and body-positivity advocate, felt like a weirdo, an outlier—like she was the only one experiencing issues with her body and with food. She grew up in a family with two sisters who were "very tiny and kind of frail," and a mother who was so thin her doctors would comment on it. "She would say all the time how she just doesn't think about food, and she would 'forget' to eat," Taussig says of her mother. Taussig never forgot to eat, though; she had a hearty appetite, especially in adolescence, when she was growing rapidly and came home from school ravenous every day. "I think there was a good month when I would make myself an entire casserole dish of custard and just eat the whole thing" as an after-school snack, she says. Though she has always lived in a smaller body, she was still "rounder and softer" than her sisters and mother, so she felt out of place.

Taussig also has paralyzed legs and severe scoliosis, and she uses a wheelchair, so she never saw herself reflected in the cultural standard of beauty. She remembers what it was like to flip through magazines as a teenager: "I'm just comparing myself to all of the images of what I'm seeing as beautiful and desirable, and I'm none of those things." So for a time she restricted her eating, thinking that would help her attain the size and shape that she saw idealized in those magazines. Of course, it never did—it resulted only in the typical swings from restriction to fuck-it-all eating and back again. More important, though, it never resulted in feeling like she was beautiful, that she was enough, or that she belonged. "No amount of restriction would make my body transform into this ideal image, because my body was always going to be paralyzed," Taussig says. So she sank into a deep shame about her body, feeling she would never measure up. "When you're experiencing something and you think you're the only one experiencing it, inherently it feels like, 'This is just me—why can't I figure it out like everybody else?'" she says.

That all changed when she discovered disability studies in graduate school. For the first time, Taussig found she wasn't alone in experiencing body shame. "To realize there are reasons, logical reasons, for you to feel that way—this didn't just come out of you, there's a whole history shaping this for a whole group of people—it's amazing how powerful that is," she says. "Just like #MeToo. I guess that's something we're seeing all over lately—the power of 'me, too.'" For Taussig, that sense of being part of something—of knowing that other people have had the same experiences, and that there are structural reasons for that—was revolutionary.

I had a similar experience when I started learning about disordered eating during my training to become a dietitian. Suddenly I became aware that all these feelings and behaviors I'd struggled to put words to for a decade had a name and fit into a framework. I felt so seen, so understood. I finally realized that I wasn't uniquely broken and weird, and that I was part of this huge group of people who've struggled with the same issues. It was liberating. There's something incredibly powerful about naming something, about having a concept or a term to describe what you're going through—because if people are talking about it and naming it, then it exists in the world, and it's something that other people have experienced, too.

It means you're not alone.

"I know there are a lot of rotten things about the internet and what it's done to us as people," Taussig says. "But one of the most amazing, magical gifts is being a part of communities of people that you wouldn't have been able to join or collaborate with otherwise." Thanks to the internet, she found and connected with a community of other disability activists, then with the body-positive community. And she's amazed at the overlaps among these communities: "We're identifying structures that have shaped our perceptions of our bodies, and together we're disassembling that structure and using our voices to make a lot of noise and change that story, change that narrative. It's been a huge gift for me."

After struggling for several years with intense weight stigma and internalized shame, a participant named Lisa in my intuitive eating online course found similar hope in online connections with people in the fat-acceptance community. Lisa had lived in a small body until she was twenty-eight, when the depression and anxiety she'd been suffering since childhood finally got diagnosed and she went on medications that significantly improved her mental health—but also caused rapid weight gain. In a matter of a few years she was in a much larger body, and now identifies as fat.

"As you can imagine," Lisa recalls, "this was quite difficult to deal with in the culture we're in." Her mother started saying mean things about her body. Her partner stopped being physically affectionate. Her friends began making fatphobic comments, couched as "concern" for her health. Lisa experienced a similar shift in treatment from her health-care providers: "Suddenly I wasn't prescribed what helped anymore, but [instead] was told to lose weight," she says. "Even my therapist kept hinting at how 'unhealthy' my lifestyle was," despite the fact that the weight gain had been caused by the psychiatric medications, not by any change in Lisa's "lifestyle."

"That led to constant rumination about how I could lose weight, but nothing worked," she says. "I tried eating as little as possible during the day, but then of course ended up bingeing. That led to a full-blown binge-eating disorder." The fact that Lisa was getting so much stigma for her weight yet could do nothing to change it pushed her into a deep depression with suicidal thoughts,* despite remaining on the meds that had been so helpful to her mental health in the past. "I felt completely worthless and unloved," she says. "I think losing the support of medical professionals—who had so far played such a big role in pulling me out of depression and anxiety—was a real shock and extremely stigmatizing. It also contributed to the hopelessness I felt. Who would I turn to? Suicide did seem like the only way out—I seemed to have lost all the support that previously kept me stable."

Thankfully, things started to change for Lisa when she reached out to someone she followed on Twitter who was vocal about fat acceptance. "They told me that fat people can be anything, even be happy. That I deserved love and support no matter my size. That my 'health' was no one's business," she says. They also recommended that Lisa check out my podcast, and she did. Soon she joined my online course, and connecting with others in the course community helped her see she wasn't the only one struggling with feelings of unworthiness about her body. "Starting the course and talking with the people in the group slowly but steadily made me realize a lot of helpful and important things: I am not alone. I am worthy. I actually have an eating disorder," she says. The group also helped her find and start working with a new therapist who specializes in Health At Every Size. And Lisa continued to educate herself about intuitive eating and HAES, the science behind these practices, the social-justice issues around body size, and the toxic effects of weight stigma.

"Slowly I became able to identify the stigmatizing actions and words of others as what they really are: a reflection of their discriminatory attitudes toward fat people, not a reflection of

---

* If you are experiencing suicidal thoughts, call the National Suicide Prevention Lifeline at 800-273-8255 (United States) or visit Befrienders at befrienders.org (worldwide).

my worth," Lisa says. "I started pushing back against my partner and demanded that he work on his internalized fatphobia. I started countering my mom's comments with snarky responses, or just ignored them." She describes this as "an incredibly hard, empowering, life-changing path," with ups and downs but ultimately leading toward liberation. "It is a movement I am proud to be a part of, and I want to keep learning," Lisa says. "It is also an exhausting battle and struggle against almost everyone I know in my offline life. More often than not, I feel too tired to fight it. But I know I want to stop letting people treat me badly because of my weight, and I know I want to become more vocal and active to speak out against fatphobia for others." Connecting with this anti-diet community has helped Lisa realize she's not alone in struggling with weight stigma, and that it's not an isolated, individual issue—it's a social and cultural one.

Even professionals in the anti-diet field need community to help us do the hard work of changing the culture. "It's so important to find a community of other Health At Every Size professionals, either in person or online, so that you have someone who gets it—because I think it can definitely be frustrating if you feel like you're alone," says Jennifer Rollin, a psychotherapist and eating-disorder specialist in private practice. "And I've certainly felt this way before—you're the lone person in a group of professionals who believes in this approach." Truly, sometimes being an anti-diet health-care provider can feel like shouting into the wind. But when we connect with other providers likewise working to dismantle diet culture, we can support one another and recharge our batteries.

For health-and-wellness professionals as well as for everyone else, the community you surround yourself with can make or break your ability to recover from diet culture. Kylie Mitchell, founder of the food-and-lifestyle blog *immaEATthat*, was in the midst of her own eating disorder when she signed up to study dietetics, where she quickly discovered the *wrong* kind of community: "Half my class was super disordered, too, and all my teachers were on diets," she remembers. Unsurprisingly, that environment exacerbated her eating disorder. "If I'd been in a different mind-set, I could have used all the nutrition information that I was learning as a tool to help myself take care of my body," Mitchell says. "But at the time it was just a weapon to harm myself and to take me more and more into my eating disorder."

Eventually Mitchell found her way to recovery—a winding path that involved getting into therapy, getting married, and getting so fed up with her disordered behaviors that she decided she couldn't spend one more second berating herself for eating a cupcake as an afternoon snack. Moving into solid recovery led her to start working in the eating-disorder field—and that's where she found a community of people to whom she could truly open up. "It was just so healing getting to talk to other dietitians about what I was struggling with," says Mitchell, "and about what I'd struggled with more severely in the past—just to be open and feel like I had a safe space." Instead of being a tool for her eating disorder, her career as a dietitian is now a source of healing.

Seeing What's Possible

When I moved to New York City in 2004, I had no idea people took the subway to the beach. I spent my days in office towers and my nights in brownstones and brick apartment buildings, and during my first few winters there were days when I never saw the sun. I'd been to Coney Island to watch the Mermaid Parade and eat at a famous pizza place called Totonno's, but I never considered swimming there or walking on the beach; I'd heard too many horror stories about polluted water and needles in the sand. Not until several years later, when my friends Alex and

Pervaiz—fellow food writers and beach lovers—started talking about a cool new taco shack in Rockaway Beach, did it occur to me that the latter was not just a Ramones song. We went for the tacos and fell in love with the Rockaways, with the beach and the dive-y Irish bars and the fascinating mix of hipsters and surfers and old-timers. Alex and Pervaiz had introduced me to my favorite escape.

We all need friends like that—friends who help us see things differently. Who take us to places where we can look up at the sky and see the sun, hear the crash of the ocean, feel the salty air on our skin and taste it on our lips. We need people who can help us remember there's a big world beyond our usual routines.

And we need people who can remind us there's life beyond diet culture. That's what an anti-diet community can do for you.

"It was really nice to see people be like, 'Actually it's OK to be fat,'" says Caleb Luna, a writer, activist, and PhD candidate who studies the relationship between bodies and discourse. Now a vocal member of the fat-acceptance movement, Luna grew up in a family that—like most families in diet culture—did *not* believe it was OK to be fat. Luna, whose pronouns are *they* and *them*, was taken to see a nutritionist when they were around twelve or thirteen, because their family believed their weight couldn't possibly be healthy. "I didn't really follow the nutritionist's plan," they say, explaining that this rebellion was a way of pushing back against the weight stigma they felt from their family. "I think because there was so much anxiety around my body size, I was afraid to validate that as a legitimate source of concern."

Luna was introduced to the fat-acceptance movement when their best friend, who also identifies as fat, recommended the book *Fat!So?* by Marilyn Wann. Soon Luna tumbled down the rabbit hole of online fat-acceptance resources. It was a revelation. "I was able to find so many fat-positive blogs and see fat people doing different things with their bodies—having active social and sexual and romantic lives, dressing fashionably, and [being] popular and loved and all these things I never felt I had access to as a fat person," they say. They also found it extraordinarily healing to witness fat people enjoying food without shame, since their own enjoyment of food had been such a point of contention in childhood. "That was really, really, really game changing for me," Luna says.

In a culture that portrays fatness as inherently unhealthy, undesirable, and emblematic of moral failure (with all the racist and sexist baggage bound up in those views), it's a radical paradigm shift to learn to see larger bodies as worthy, lovable, and desirable. Changing how you relate to body size refutes everything diet culture teaches us. And it's helpful not just for people who identify as fat—it's helpful for everyone, of *all* sizes. Surrounding yourself with evidence that people in larger bodies are worthy of basic human rights and of having fulfilling, kick-ass lives helps deprogram the diet-culture bullshit we've been brainwashed to believe. It helps reduce internalized weight stigma—which pretty much everyone struggles with in this culture, and which harms your well-being regardless of body size.[1]

Lest you worry that this "glorifies obesity," as the internet trolls love to say, recall Chapter 5's evidence that weight *stigma* is a bigger risk to people's health than weight itself and what they eat. Denigrating people's bodies has never improved anyone's well-being. Our culture has been tearing down larger bodies for more than 150 years now, and where has that gotten us? Epidemic levels of disordered eating, body loathing, and fatphobia, which have never been shown to help individuals—or society as a whole—be any healthier or happier. On the contrary, weight stigma makes people less likely to engage in physical activity or so-called "healthy eating"; more likely to struggle with their mental health; and more likely to develop a host of chronic diseases and conditions they might escape if our society didn't treat them like garbage. With all the weight stigma that's baked into diet culture, larger bodies could *use* some glorifying. And when we lift them up as beautiful, worthy, powerful, and human, we lift up people of *all* sizes. We help create a more just and peaceful world for everybody in every kind of body.

Coping IRL

Creating an anti-diet online community is clutch, but what about the people you know in real life? As covered in Chapter 7, setting boundaries around diet talk with your friends and family is essential for your healing, but it can also be tricky. There are profound benefits to life beyond diet culture, but you may also feel disconnected from the people around you when you first start rejecting the Life Thief and stop participating in its rituals. It's easy to feel left out when everyone in your life is bonding over restrictive practices such as "clean eating," Whole30, keto, or whatever form the Wellness Diet takes next. When you stop pursuing weight loss and the Wellness Diet, you leave a community behind—the community of diet culture.

"Any kind of restrictive diet creates a community," says religious scholar Alan Levinovitz. "You're a vegetarian or you're a Paleo eater, and that creates solidarity." When you're engaged in diet culture, you're participating in a group with its own rituals, its own rules—and so many people hunger for groups like that today, particularly in the secular world. "As religious eating rituals disappear and as religion itself recedes as a source of authority on what we ought to do for our health, it seems to me a logical step to think that dietary practices are helping to fill that in," Levinovitz says. So be aware that distancing yourself from diet culture might feel like losing your religion.

Not only that, but when you're surrounded by people still invested in diet culture, it's hard not to get sucked back in. You might find yourself starting to envy friends' "healthy lifestyles"—

even if part of you can see those behaviors as disordered eating, orthorexia, compulsive exercise, or other strains of diet culture. You might feel body shame when you compare yourself with family members still on the diet train—even though you know they'll be weight-cycling for years to come, and that whatever "success" they're having now is short-lived and comes at a steep cost. Despite everything you now know about diet culture, it can still feel seductive when you're in a community that's mired in it.

It's helpful to identify a few people you trust who can have your back in the fight against diet culture. That way, you can face potentially triggering situations knowing you have an ally. "My husband and I started doing this thing when I was recovering where anytime we heard a diet-mentality comment—whether we were at a restaurant, grocery store, or holiday family event—we would just mutter under our breath to each other, 'EDB,' [which stands for] eating-disorder behavior," Kylie Mitchell says. "That was always really helpful to call it out for what it was. It might be, you know, Aunt Susie or whatever saying some comment she thinks is harmless, but it really can affect those with eating disorders." Having someone close by who can help you recognize those EDBs can help you avoid getting all turned around and thinking you should try whatever diet-culture behavior is being shoved in your face. Even if you're not physically with your anti-diet ally, you can call or text them for support. (Never underestimate the power of a well-timed eye-roll emoji from someone who gets it!)

Of course, not all of your loved ones will be in your corner right away—it can take a lot of difficult conversations, sometimes over the course of years, to bring some people around. "It's very difficult when you have such close relationships already," says Evette Dionne, the editor in chief of Bitch Media, who's had a long road to getting her mother on board with her body-positive, anti-diet stance. "She and I have been in relationship for twenty-eight years, and now I'm shifting what that looks like. That is really scary terrain. It's very difficult when you've been in a relationship for so long to now say, 'Hey, I want to have a conversation about what you said about my body,' or, 'When you say that to me, it hurts me'—particularly when you allowed it to go on for so long because you didn't know any different." People often experience friction in relationships when they first start having these kinds of conversations, Dionne points out, and that can cause discomfort that makes them stop pushing for change. But if you can work through that discomfort, it opens up the possibility of having the relationship grow and evolve, so that it becomes nourishing and supportive for *both* parties. "I am trying to get to a point where I have the courage to continue to push forward," Dionne says.

Some people in your life may be genuinely unsafe to keep engaging with—those who are outright malicious or abusive, even if they don't intend to be, because they can't empathize with your point of view or lack the capacity to change. Sometimes you have to do a lot of soul-searching to know when it's time to let go of a relationship with someone who isn't able to grow in the ways you need, as opposed to understanding when it's just going to take time and effort for the person to change. "There's a difference between being in a relationship with people who are toxic—there's no redemption there, no way of salvaging that relationship—and being in a relationship with someone who has given you so much and there's just one or two things that they really have to work their way through," Dionne says. It's important to consider the relationship as a whole, and the effect on your life of leaving it—because of course you need a support system. "If I completely disown everyone in my immediate family in my all-white town because we have different beliefs, then I have no village—I have no one to rely on, I have no community," Dionne says. "Is it worth that? That's something all people have to weigh for themselves."

It's also worth bearing in mind that everyone has different access to knowledge and information—and when it comes to knowing about the harms of diet culture, right now that's the province of only a small percentage of the population (that is, cool people like you). "That's why I always ask people to make space for grace instead of condemning people," Dionne says. "You have to make space for people to be imperfect. Just allow people the space, the time, and the energy to grow in their thinking, to evolve in their mind-set, to shift in their behaviors. There's this impatience for people to change overnight, and that just doesn't happen." For Dionne and her mom the shift has happened, but it has required a lot more than just one conversation: "We've been having these conversations for two years," she says. "I've been asking her not to make comments about my body for *two years*, and now we're in a place where that can happen."

It's certainly easier when you're starting a new relationship from scratch, because you get to put your anti-diet values—and any other values that are important to you—front and center. "Now I'm at a point in my life where I'm very conscious of creating relationships with people," Dionne says. "I have consciousness around, well, *Is the person triggering to me or not? Does the person have ideas that mirror mine, or do they have oppressive behaviors?*" She views creating new relationships with people as a choice, and she deliberately seeks out people who support her body-positive beliefs. That's something you can consider doing from here on as well.

Viral Change

Before you overhaul your entire friend group in search of new pals who already get it, know that spreading the anti-diet message to others in your existing network—even if they seem resistant at first—can have huge ripple effects in terms of social change. That's because innovations, from new agricultural practices to new technological devices, are spread through social networks (even those that existed before social media). Specifically, a small minority of people—the innovators and early adopters in any given network, otherwise known as the cool people—pick up the new innovations first; others then follow suit because they see those in the cultural vanguard doing it and become convinced it's the smart thing to do.[2]

The anti-diet movement, including the practices of Health At Every Size and intuitive eating, follows a similar pattern. "You learn about it from your colleagues or your friends," says Fiona Willer, a HAES dietitian, author, and lecturer based in Queensland, Australia. "The benefits are communicated through those social networks, and it spreads like a virus. So in that way, I've talked about HAES being like an iPhone." And as with technology, the cool people can have a disproportionate impact on the dissemination of HAES by talking about it with everyone they know. "It means we need to keep talking," Willer says. "Talk to everyone—anyone. The person in the line at the shops. Just get it out there, because it is viral."

It can help to start with the people you're most likely to convince. The ones who consider themselves socially conscious. The Facebook friend who's constantly sharing stories about immigration rights and police brutality. The aunt who always urges you to canvass for progressive candidates with her. The neighbors down the street with the protest signs in their window. These people care about issues of social justice and are already invested in making the world a more equitable place. So talk to them about diet culture, about the discrimination and stigma it creates against larger-bodied people. Talk to them about how the Wellness Diet harms our well-being, and how the "obesity epidemic" is a myth created by diet-industry allies to sell more weight-loss drugs. Talk to them about how the food-activist movement is built on a foundation of "obesity epidemic" rhetoric—which itself is built on a foundation of racist and misogynistic ideas about bodies—and about how to address issues of food access without any vestiges of diet culture. Like all of us, these people will probably have some degree of resistance because of the diet-culture messages they've internalized over the years. They might even be super bought-in to the Wellness Diet right now. But their social-justice awareness also makes them more likely to eventually understand why we need to take down diet culture.

Granted, those conversations can consume a lot of emotional energy, and sometimes you don't have the bandwidth for that. Sometimes planting a seed in people's minds is enough—and in many situations you wouldn't want to undertake a long conversation about diet culture even if you had the time and energy. Sometimes people just aren't ready, leading them to debate or attack you, which feels like total garbage when you're on the receiving end of it. They generally do this because they're upset to hear that everything our culture has told them about food and bodies is a lie. And that's completely understandable.

Ten years ago, when I'd just entered the nutrition field because I wanted to help end the "obesity epidemic," I got really hot under the collar and defensive with the friend who first introduced me to Health At Every Size. Now here I am a decade later, writing a book about how great it is. So I get it. We all have our own paths out of diet culture. The people in your life will need time and space to react when they learn about the Life Thief. That's another good place for setting boundaries: when you tell people about diet culture and they get worked up, you can walk away from the conversation. You needn't convince them in one sitting. Sometimes the best thing you can do is plant a seed by saying something tiny and quick, such as, "Actually I don't like to moralize about food," or, "I'm not an advocate of weight loss, because in my experience it does more harm than good." You never know when that seed is going to take root—when someone else's anti-diet awakening is going to happen.

There's so much potential for social change in this arena. I hope that reading this book has helped open your mind to some of the ways we can push for a more just, equitable world for people in *all* bodies. This change can come from every corner, and it can take lots of creative forms. As Willer explains, anyone can be a part of it—even those who've been deeply invested in diet culture. "All the people putting effort into trying to make larger bodies smaller—could they not design appliances to help people live fully actualized lives in the bodies that they have?" she says. "If they put that effort and their brilliant design minds into helping diverse bodies become more able to experience the world, enhance health—all the things that weight loss is sold as the solution to—with the bodies that they have now," that would truly revolutionize the health-care industry and our world.

Reclaiming Your Life

If there's one thing I hope you'll take from this book, it's this: You don't have to spend all your time and energy worrying about food and your body. You *can* have more mental space to do your work, take care of yourself, spend time with your loved ones, and answer your calling. To, you know, change the world. People are capable of doing incredible things with the time and energy they reclaim when they stop dieting. Things like starting their own businesses, advocating for social justice and human rights, going back to school to pursue their dreams, finding supportive partners who love them unconditionally, and raising their kids to feel good about their bodies and trust their instincts with food. Things that help build a better life for themselves and others.

It's time we all had the opportunity to do these things. It's time for a sea change. There's so much at stake: our time, money, well-being, happiness—and, above all, our fundamental human rights. Diet culture has already stolen the lives of millions. We can't let it continue. We can't let the Life Thief claim another generation, under the guise of "health" and "wellness" and "empowerment."

The movement to dismantle diet culture is a movement for social justice, for equal rights, for people in bodies of all shapes and sizes. And this movement is on the right side of history, just like every other movement to end oppression and grant equal rights to people of diverse ethnicities, genders, sexual orientations, and all the other identities that make up humanity's rich tapestry. The more we spread the anti-diet message, the better off everyone—in *every* kind of body—is going to be.

We all have a role to play in making this change happen. It starts with reclaiming your life.

Acknowledgments

I'd been circling around the ideas in this book for more than ten years, but I was only able to bring it into the world thanks to my own healing from diet culture—and thanks to the support and inspiration I've received from the activists, writers, scholars, health-care providers, and others who came before me in this anti-diet movement. To Evelyn Tribole, Elyse Resch, Deb Burgard, Lindo Bacon, Lisa Pearl, Chevese Turner, Virgie Tovar, Lisa DuBreuil, Isabel Foxen Duke, Sonya Renee Taylor, Ragen Chastain, Marilyn Wann, Bill Fabrey, the late Joanne Ikeda, and countless others in the Health At Every Size and fat-positive communities, thank you for blazing this trail by naming the problems with our culture's view of weight and bringing an alternative paradigm to life. I'm honored to be walking in your footsteps. I also owe so much of my recovery to therapy, and specifically to the fact that fifteen years ago I stumbled into MK as my therapist—who, despite not specializing in eating disorders, gave me the compassion and the emotional self-care skills I needed to heal my relationship with food and my body.

I'm deeply grateful to Kelly Diels, feminist marketing coach extraordinaire, for helping me come up with the organizing metaphor of the Life Thief, and for seeing the book in me and giving me the push I needed to put together a proposal.

My wonderful agent, Brettne Bloom, believed in this idea from day one and offered wisdom and encouragement every step of the way. Thanks as well to her assistant at The Book Group, Hallie Schaeffer, whose thoughtful input on the proposal helped hone my vision of diet culture, particularly of the Wellness Diet.

To the whole team at Little, Brown Spark, thank you for "getting" this book right away. (In our pitch meeting I felt so understood that I left my body for a second and did a little dance in my mind.) Throughout the publishing process my editor, Marisa Vigilante, gave me the kind of insightful and supportive feedback every writer dreams of, and helped amplify my social-justice message at every turn. Publisher Tracy Behar welcomed me with open arms to her new Spark list. Ian Straus, Jules Horbachevsky, Jess Chun, and Karen Landry did a masterly job of shepherding this book along and helping get it into readers' hands. Copyeditor Allan Fallow polished my prose beautifully (and saved me from repeating the word *incredible* 10,000 times).

A huge thanks to my longtime friend Karen Rose Stave for her careful fact-checking and support in making this book the best it could be. Many thanks as well to Alex Van Buren for reading the manuscript when it was still very much under construction and helping me put up the essential support beams, and to Maria Paredes and Sand Chang for helping me think through some important passages. Dan Engber planted the seed of the HAES paradigm for me ten years ago. Conversations over meals with Fiona Sutherland, Rebecca Scritchfield, Marci Evans, Jamie Aderski, Joy Cox, and Julie Duffy Dillon—and podcast interviews with dozens of other friends and colleagues in this movement—helped me hone my perspective and stay fired up to smash diet culture in all its forms.

Speaking of interviews, I'm deeply indebted to all of my sources for sharing their stories and expertise throughout this book. Your willingness to open up about what were often painful experiences might just be saving the life of someone else who's going through the same thing right now. Thank you for your generosity and vulnerability.

I never would've found the time to write this book if it weren't for my team at Food Psych Programs, who helped keep my business running smoothly so that I could turn off my devices and concentrate. Ashley Seruya and Vincci Tsui created beautiful social-media posts and show notes for my podcast; along with Ashley Sobel, they also provided incomparable research assistance for the book. Kimmie Singh stepped in during Vincci's maternity leave to keep things running seamlessly. Julianne Wotasik and SJ Thompson helped me stay in touch with the outside world and made sure my in-box didn't explode. Mike Lalonde kept my podcast coming out and sounding amazing every week. Vincci, Kierra McClellan, and Meghan Cichy transcribed it, so that people who couldn't hear it could still benefit from its messages.

None of my work would have been possible without my family, to whom I'm endlessly grateful for helping me become the person I am. To my sister, thanks for always having my back. You've been an incredible friend and sounding board throughout the process of writing this book, and throughout life. And I wouldn't be here today—literally or figuratively—without my parents, who "published" my first "books" by dictation before I could hold a pen. Mom and Dad, thank you for always supporting my dreams, teaching me the importance of social justice, and never holding back with the big words.

And finally, to my wonderful husband, thank you for giving me the strength and the space to make this book a reality. Not only did you cook all the meals, do all the errands and dishes, and listen to all the worries of a first-time author for two years straight, you also read countless drafts and gave me thoughtful feedback that sharpened my writing every time. You handled it all with remarkable grace and managed to keep me smiling and laughing along the way. I love you and am so lucky I get to go through life by your side. Thank you for loving me.

Resources

Here's a list of some of my favorite resources—websites, blogs, books, podcasts, social-media accounts, online communities, and more—to help support you in life beyond diet culture. Of course, I can't be responsible for the contents of any publications other than my own, so I can't guarantee they'll be 100 percent trigger-free. But the resources on this list have helped my clients and/or informed my own anti-diet journey—and I have a feeling they'll help you on yours, too.

Books

Big Girl: How I Gave Up Dieting and Got a Life by Kelsey Miller

The Body Is Not an Apology: The Power of Radical Self-Love by Sonya Renee Taylor

Body Positive Power: Because Life Is Already Happening and You Don't Need Flat Abs to Live It by Megan Jayne Crabbe

Body Respect: What Conventional Health Books Get Wrong, Leave Out, and Just Plain Fail to Understand About Weight by Lindo Bacon and Lucy Aphramor

Body of Truth: How Science, History, and Culture Drive Our Obsession with Weight—and What We Can Do About It by Harriet Brown

The Diet Survivor's Handbook: 60 Lessons in Eating, Acceptance and Self-Care by Judith Matz and Ellen Frankel

The Eating Instinct: Food Culture, Body Image, and Guilt in America by Virginia Sole-Smith

Embody: Learning to Love Your Unique Body (and Quiet That Critical Voice!) by Connie Sobczak

Every Body Yoga: Let Go of Fear, Get on the Mat, Love Your Body by Jessamyn Stanley

Fat Shame: Stigma and the Fat Body in American Culture by Amy Erdman Farrell

Fat!So?: Because You Don't Have to Apologize for Your Size by Marilyn Wann

Fearing the Black Body: The Racial Origins of Fat Phobia by Sabrina Strings

The F*ck-It Diet: Eating Should Be Easy by Caroline Dooner

The Gluten Lie: And Other Myths About What You Eat by Alan Levinovitz

The Intuitive Eating Workbook: Ten Principles for Nourishing a Healthy Relationship with Food by Evelyn Tribole and Elyse Resch

Just Eat It: How Intuitive Eating Can Help You Get Your Shit Together Around Food by Laura Thomas

Lessons from the Fat-o-sphere: Quit Dieting and Declare a Truce with Your Body by Kate Harding and Marianne Kirby

Let It Out: A Journey Through Journaling by Katie Dalebout

Shrill: Notes from a Loud Woman by Lindy West

Things No One Will Tell Fat Girls: A Handbook for Unapologetic Living by Jes Baker

What's Wrong with Fat? by Abigail C. Saguy

You Have the Right to Remain Fat by Virgie Tovar

Websites and Blogs

My site: christyharrison.com

The Adipositivity Project: adipositivity.com

Association for Size Diversity and Health (ASDAH): sizediversityand health.org

Beauty Redefined: beautyredefined.org

Be Nourished: benourished.org

The Body Is Not an Apology: thebodyisnotanapology.com

Curvy Yoga: curvyyoga.com

Dances with Fat: danceswithfat.org

Dare to Not Diet: daretonotdiet.wordpress.com

Everyday Feminism: everydayfeminism.com

ImmaEATthat: immaeatthat.com

Isabel Foxen Duke: isabelfoxenduke.com

Lindo Bacon, PhD: lindobacon.com
Melissa A. Fabello, PhD: melissafabello.com
The Militant Baker: themilitantbaker.com
Representation Matters: representationmatters.me
Virgie Tovar: virgietovar.com

Podcasts

Food Psych (my podcast) — christyharrison.com/foodpsych
Body Kindness: bodykindnessbook.com/podcast
The Bodylove Project: jessihaggerty.com/blppodcast
Dietitians Unplugged: dietitiansunplugged.libsyn.com
Don't Salt My Game: laurathomasphd.co.uk/category/podcast
Fearless Rebelle Radio: summerinnanen.com/frr
Fresh Out the Cocoon: freshoutthecocoon.com/blogs/news
The F*ck-It Diet Radio: thefuckitdiet.com/tag/podcast
Love, Food: juliedillonrd.com/lovefoodpodcast
She's All Fat: shesallfatpod.com
Your Body, Your Brand: bodybrandpod.com

Social Media

Christy Harrison: @chr1styharrison on Instagram and Twitter
Lindo Bacon: @lindobaconx on Twitter and Facebook
Jes Baker: @themilitantbaker on Instagram and Twitter
Megan Jayne Crabbe: @bodyposipanda on Instagram and @bodypo
    sipanda_ on Twitter
Isabel Foxen Duke: @isabelfoxenduke on Instagram and Twitter
Caleb Luna: @chairbreaker on Instagram and @tummyfuq on Twitter
Meredith Noble: @madeonagenerousplan on Instagram and @gener
    ousplan on Twitter
Fiona Sutherland: @themindfuldietitian on Instagram and @Fion
    aBodyPosAus on Twitter
Rebekah Taussig: @sitting_pretty on Instagram
Sonya Renee Taylor: @sonyareneetaylor on Instagram and @Sonyare
    neepoet on Twitter
Virgie Tovar: @virgietovar on Instagram and Twitter

Online Courses and Communities

Intuitive Eating Fundamentals: christyharrison.com/course

Body Kindness Spiral Up Club: bodykindnessbook.com/spiralup

The Intuitive Eating Moms Club: intuitiveeatingmoms.com

Lose Hate Not Weight Babecamp: virgietovar.com/babecamp

No More Weighting: The Body Trust® E-Course: benourished.org/
no-more-weighting-the-body-trust-ecourse

PCOS and Food Peace: pcosandfoodpeace.com

UNTRAPPED course: untrapped.com.au

Anti-Diet Health-Care Providers

Christy Harrison: christyharrison.com

Be Nourished: benourished.org

Kathleen Bishop, LCSW: bodypeaceliberation.com

The Certified Intuitive Eating Counselors Directory: intuitiveeating
.org/certified-counselors

Sand Chang, PhD: sandchang.com

Carmen Cool, MA, LPC: carmencool.com

Lisa DuBreuil, LICSW: lisadubreuil.com

Marci Evans, MS, RD, CEDRD-S: marcird.com

Dana Falsetti: danafalsetti.com

Kristy Fassio: rooted-heart.com

Aaron Flores, RDN: bvmrd.com

Lilia Graue, MD, LMFT: liliagrauemd.com

The HAES Community Registry: haescommunity.com/search

Jessi Haggerty, RDN, CPT: jessihaggerty.com

Sarah Harry, RYT: bodypositiveaustralia.com.au

Rachel Millner, PsyD: rachelmillner.com

Kylie Mitchell, MPH, RDN: immaeatthat.com/nutrition-counseling

Amy Pershing, LMSW, ACSW: thebodywiseprogram.com

Recovered Living: recoveredliving.com

Jennifer Rollin, MSW, LCSW-C: jenniferrollin.com

Rebecca Scritchfield, MA, RDN: bodykindnessbook.com

Victoria Welsby: fiercefatty.com

Fiona Willer, AdvAPD: healthnotdiets.com

Notes

The following publications are valuable references, but most of them still contain some fatphobic language and/or potentially triggering details—even some of the books and articles critiquing the diet industry and the "war on obesity." That's how deeply entrenched diet culture is. Read them with a critical eye, and if you're struggling with disordered-eating or exercise behaviors, proceed with caution or leave them on the shelf.

Introduction

1. See, for example, Lindo Bacon and Lucy Aphramor, "Weight Science: Evaluating the Evidence for a Paradigm Shift," *Nutrition Journal* 10, no. 9 (January 2011).
2. Tracy L. Tylka et al., "The Weight-Inclusive Versus Weight-Normative Approach to Health: Evaluating the Evidence for Prioritizing Well-Being over Weight Loss," *Journal of Obesity* 2014, Article ID 983495 (2014).
3. Traci Mann et al., "Medicare's Search for Effective Obesity Treatments: Diets Are Not the Answer," *American Psychologist* 62, no. 3 (April 2007).
4. Marketdata LLC, "The U.S. Weight Loss and Diet Control Market: A Market Research Analysis," 15th edition (February 2019).
5. E. W. Diemer et al., "Beyond the Binary: Differences in Eating Disorder Prevalence by Gender Identity in a Transgender Sample," *Transgender Health* 3, no. 1 (January 2018): 17–23.

Chapter 1: The Roots of Diet Culture

1. Susan E. Hill, *Eating to Excess: The Meaning of Gluttony and the Fat Body in the Ancient World* (ABC-CLIO, 2011).
2. Hillel Schwartz, *Never Satisfied: A Cultural History of Diets, Fantasies, and Fat* (Free Press, 1986).
3. P. J. Brown, "Culture and the Evolution of Obesity," in D. Kulick and A. Meneley, eds., *Fat: The Anthropology of an Obsession* (Jeremy P. Tarcher/Penguin, 2005).
4. P. J. Brown and M. Konner, "An Anthropological Perspective on Obesity," *Annals of the New York Academy of Sciences* 499 (1987): 29–46.

5. Louise Foxcroft, *Calories & Corsets: A History of Dieting over 2,000 Years* (Profile Books, 2011).

6. M. Bradley, "Obesity, Corpulence, and Emaciation in Roman Art," *Papers of the British School at Rome* 79 (2011): 1–41.

7. Jana Evans Braziel and Kathleen LeBesco, eds., *Bodies Out of Bounds: Fatness and Transgression* (University of California Press, 2001).

8. Hippocrates, *Hippocratic Writings* (Penguin UK, 2005). Note that some writings attributed to Hippocrates were most likely written by his students and followers. See J. Jouanna and N. Allies, "Dietetics in Hippocratic Medicine: Definition, Main Problems, Discussion," in Philip Van Der Eijk, ed., *Greek Medicine from Hippocrates to Galen: Selected Papers* (Brill, 2012).

9. Bradley, "Obesity," 2011.

10. Jouanna and Allies, "Dietetics," 2012.

11. *Ibid.*

12. R. Earle, " 'If You Eat Their Food…': Diets and Bodies in Early Colonial Spanish America," *American Historical Review* 115, no. 3 (2010): 688–713. Thanks to Gloria Lucas of Nalgona Positivity Pride for alerting me to this research.

13. For example, male conquistadors saw their beards as a gift from God, and were horrified by the mostly beardless faces of the indigenous men (Earle, "If You Eat Their Food," 2010).

14. Kenneth E. Hendrickson III, ed., "Slater, Samuel (1768–1835)," *The Encyclopedia of the Industrial Revolution in World History,* vol. 3 (Rowman & Littlefield, 2014).

15. Schwartz, *Never Satisfied,* 1986.

16. B. Dorsey, *Reforming Men and Women: Gender in the Antebellum City* (Cornell University Press, 2002).

17. Schwartz, *Never Satisfied,* 1986.

18. *Ibid.*

19. Jonathan Rees, "Industrialization and Urbanization in the United States, 1880–1929," *Oxford Research Encyclopedia of American History,* http://americanhistory.oxfordre.com/view/10.1093/acrefore/9780199329175.001.0001/acrefore-9780199329175-e-327.

20. Laura Fraser, *Losing It: False Hopes and Fat Profits in the Diet Industry* (Plume, 1997).

21. Amy Erdman Farrell, *Fat Shame: Stigma and the Fat Body in American Culture* (New York University Press, 2011).

22. Sabrina Strings, *Fearing the Black Body: The Racial Origins of Fat Phobia* (New York University Press, 2019).

23. *Ibid.*

24. Farrell, *Fat Shame,* 2011.

25. Greg Critser, "Legacy of a Fat Man," *The Guardian,* September 19, 2003, https://www.theguardian.com/theguardian/2003/sep/20/weekend7.weekend1.

26. R. Bivins and H. Marland, "Weighting for Health: Management, Measurement and Self-Surveillance in the Modern Household," *Social History of Medicine* 29, no. 4 (2016): 757–80.

27. William Banting, *Letter on Corpulence: Addressed to the Public* (Harrison, 1864). [No relation.]

28. Schwartz, *Never Satisfied*, 1986.

29. Fraser, *Losing It*, 1997.

30. National Museum of American Illustration, "Charles Dana Gibson: 1867–1944," https://americanillustration.org/project/charles-dana-gibson/.

31. Fraser, *Losing It*, 1997.

32. Farrell, *Fat Shame*, 2011.

33. Fraser, *Losing It*, 1997.

34. Helen Zoe Veit, *Modern Food, Moral Food: Self-Control, Science, and the Rise of Modern American Eating in the Early Twentieth Century* (University of North Carolina Press, 2013).

35. Naomi Wolf, *The Beauty Myth: How Images of Beauty Are Used Against Women* (William Morrow, 1991).

36. Farrell, *Fat Shame*, 2011.

37. *Ibid.*

38. Peter N. Stearns, *Fat History: Bodies and Beauty in the Modern West* (New York University Press, 1997).

39. Schwartz, *Never Satisfied*, 1986.

40. Sindya N. Bhanoo, "Study Suggests BMI Scale Is Weighted Against African Americans," *Washington Post*, April 14, 2009, http://www.washingtonpost.com/wp-dyn/content/article/2009/04/13/AR2009041301823.html.

41. Schwartz, *Never Satisfied*, 1986.

42. K. M. Flegal et al., "Association of All-Cause Mortality with Overweight and Obesity Using Standard Body Mass Index Categories: A Systematic Review and Meta-analysis," *JAMA* 309, no. 1 (January 2, 2013): 71–82.

43. A. J. Tomiyama et al., "Misclassification of Cardiometabolic Health When Using Body Mass Index Categories in NHANES 2005–2012," *International Journal of Obesity* 40, no. 5 (2016): 883–86.

44. Schwartz, *Never Satisfied*, 1986.

45. Veit, *Modern Food*, 2013.

46. *Ibid.*

47. Schwartz, *Never Satisfied*, 1986.

48. Sander L. Gilman, *Diets and Dieting: A Cultural Encyclopedia* (Routledge, 2008); Henry Buchwald, "The History of Bariatric Surgery: My Life in Metabolic Surgery," *Bariatric Times* 12, no. 7 (2015): 12–14, http://bariatrictimes.com/the-history-of-bariatric-surgery/.

49. J. Eric Oliver, *Fat Politics: The Real Story Behind America's Obesity Epidemic* (Oxford University Press, 2005).

50. Schwartz, *Never Satisfied*, 1986; Robert D. McFadden, "Jean Nidetch, a Founder of Weight Watchers, Dies at 91," *New York Times*, April 29, 2015.

51. Schwartz, *Never Satisfied,* 1986.

52. *Ibid.*

53. Ann F. La Berge, "How the Ideology of Low Fat Conquered America," *Journal of the History of Medicine and Allied Sciences* 63, no. 2 (April 2008): 139–77.

54. National Institutes of Health (NIH), "Methods for Voluntary Weight Loss and Control," *Annals of Internal Medicine* 116, no. 11 (June 1992).

55. Bob Greene, "Oprah's Weight Loss Confession," oprah.com, January 5, 2009, https://www.oprah.com/health/oprahs-weight-loss-confession.

56. Abigail Trafford, "Losing the Weight Battle," *Washington Post,* February 7, 1995, https://www.washingtonpost.com/archive/lifestyle/wellness/1995/02/07/losing-the-weight-battle/da649449-bf3f-4bf1-a08f-f0999b0c9d31/.

57. J. Montani et al., "Weight Cycling and Cardiometabolic Risks," *Obesity Reviews* 16 (February 2015), Suppl 1: 7–18.

58. Oliver, *Fat Politics,* 2005. See also Ray Moynihan, "Obesity Task Force Linked to WHO Takes 'Millions' from Drug Firms," *BMJ* 332, no. 7555 (June 17, 2006): 1412. The IOTF has since rebranded itself as the World Obesity Federation (see https://www.worldobesity.org/who-we-are/history/).

59. Oliver, *Fat Politics,* 2005.

60. D. Mandrioli et al., "Relationship Between Research Outcomes and Risk of Bias, Study Sponsorship, and Author Financial Conflicts of Interest in Reviews of the Effects of Artificially Sweetened Beverages on Weight Outcomes: A Systematic Review of Reviews," *PLOS ONE* 11, no. 9 (September 2016): e0162198.

61. Oliver, *Fat Politics,* 2005.

62. Abigail C. Saguy, *What's Wrong with Fat?* (Oxford University Press, 2013); U.S. Bureau of Labor Statistics Inflation Calculator, https://data.bls.gov/cgi-bin/cpicalc.pl.

63. Oliver, *Fat Politics,* 2005.

64. Jeffery Sobal, "The Medicalization and Demedicalization of Obesity," in Donna Maurer and Jeffery Sobal, eds., *Eating Agendas: Food and Nutrition as Social Problems* (Walter De Gruyter, 1995).

65. Oliver, *Fat Politics,* 2005.

66. The CDC has continued adding to these maps every year, and it has since started using a yellow-orange color for the levels between blue and red.

67. Oliver, *Fat Politics,* 2005.

68. Paul Campos, Abigail Saguy, Paul Ernsberger, Eric Oliver, and Glenn Gaesser, "The Epidemiology of Overweight and Obesity: Public Health Crisis or Moral Panic?" *International Journal of Epidemiology* 35, no. 1 (February 1, 2006): 55–60.

69. Oliver, *Fat Politics,* 2005.

70. Andrew Pollack, "A.M.A. Recognizes Obesity as a Disease," *New York Times,* June 18, 2013, https://www.nytimes.com/2013/06/19/business/ama-recognizes-obesity-as-a-disease.html.

Chapter 2: A Diet by Another Name

1. Abigail C. Saguy, *What's Wrong with Fat?* (Oxford University Press, 2013).
2. D. A. Frederick et al., "Effects of Competing News Media Frames of Weight on Antifat Stigma, Beliefs About Weight and Support for Obesity-Related Public Policies," *International Journal of Obesity* 40, no. 3 (2016): 543–49; Abigail C. Saguy, David Frederick, and Kjerstin Gruys, "Reporting Risk, Producing Prejudice: How News Reporting on Obesity Shapes Attitudes About Health Risk, Policy, and Prejudice," *Social Science & Medicine* 111 (2014): 125–33; D. A. Frederick et al., "Culture, Health, and Bigotry: How Exposure to Cultural Accounts of Fatness Shape Attitudes About Health Risk, Health Policies, and Weight-Based Prejudice," *Social Science & Medicine* 165 (2016): 271–79.
3. Saguy, *What's Wrong with Fat?*, 2013.
4. Frederick et al., "Effects," 2016.
5. S. Täuber, "Moralized Health-Related Persuasion Undermines Social Cohesion," *Frontiers in Psychology* 9 (2018): 909.
6. Eric Schlosser, *Fast Food Nation: The Dark Side of the All-American Meal* (Perennial, 2001).
7. Ximena Ramos Salas, "The Ineffectiveness and Unintended Consequences of the Public Health War on Obesity," *Canadian Journal of Public Health* 106, no. 2 (February 3, 2015): e79–81.
8. Marion Nestle, *Food Politics: How the Food Industry Influences Nutrition and Health* (University of California Press, 2002).
9. Michael Pollan, *The Omnivore's Dilemma: A Natural History of Four Meals* (Penguin Books, 2006).
10. Michael Pollan, *In Defense of Food: An Eater's Manifesto* (Penguin Press, 2008).
11. Julie Guthman, *Weighing In: Obesity, Food Justice, and the Limits of Capitalism* (University of California Press, 2011).
12. Michael Pollan, *Food Rules: An Eater's Manual* (Penguin Books, 2009).
13. Saguy, *What's Wrong with Fat?*, 2013.
14. Guthman, *Weighing In*, 2011.
15. A. Fasano et al., "Prevalence of Celiac Disease in At-Risk and Not-At-Risk Groups in the United States: A Large Multicenter Study," *Archives of Internal Medicine* 163, no. 3 (February 2003): 286–92.
16. C. Boyd et al., "Psychological Features Are Important Predictors of Functional Gastrointestinal Disorders in Patients with Eating Disorders," *Scandinavian Journal of Gastroenterology* 40, no. 8 (2005): 929–35.
17. R. Satherley et al., "Disordered Eating Practices in Gastrointestinal Disorders," *Appetite* 84 (2015): 240–50.
18. J. M. Kelso, "Unproven Diagnostic Tests for Adverse Reactions to Foods," *Journal of Allergy and Clinical Immunology: In Practice* 6, no. 2 (2018): 362–65.
19. See, for example, Eliza Barclay and Allison Aubrey, "Doctors Say Changes in Wheat Do Not Explain Rise of Celiac Disease," NPR,

September 26, 2013, https://www.npr.org/sections/thesalt/2013/09/26/
226510988/doctors-say-changes-in-wheat-do-not-explain-rise-of-celiac
-disease, accessed May 9, 2018; Alan Levinovitz, "The Problem with
David Perlmutter, the *Grain Brain* Doctor," *The Cut,* June 24, 2015,
https://www.thecut.com/2015/06/problem-with-the-grain-brain
-doctor.html, accessed May 9, 2018.

20. "About the Magazine," *Clean Eating,* https://www.cleaneatingmag.com/
page/about, accessed February 6, 2018.

21. Steven Bratman, *Health Food Junkies: Overcoming the Obsession with Healthful
Eating* (Broadway Books, 2001).

22. Pixie G. Turner and Carmen E. Lefevre, "Instagram Use Is Linked to
Increased Symptoms of Orthorexia Nervosa," *Eating and Weight Disorders*
22, no. 2 (2017): 277–84.

23. S. Bratman, "Orthorexia vs. Theories of Healthy Eating," *Eating and Weight
Disorders—Studies on Anorexia, Bulimia and Obesity* 22, no. 3 (2017): 381–85.

24. Marketdata LLC, "The U.S. Weight Loss and Diet Control Market: A Market
Research Analysis," 14th edition (May 2017); Marketdata Enterprises,
"The Diet Market: Our Specialty—for 28 Years!," https://www.market
dataenterprises.com/diet-market-our-specialty/, accessed April 6, 2018.

25. John LaRosa, "Top 6 Trends for the Weight Loss Industry in 2018,"
MarketResearch.com, January 2, 2018, https://blog.marketresearch
.com/top-6-trends-for-the-weight-loss-market-in-2018.

26. Phil Wahba, "Weight Watchers Changes Name to 'WW' in Wellness
Push," *Fortune,* September 24, 2018, http://fortune.com/2018/09/24/
weight-watchers-name-change/.

27. Jasmine Hemsley and Melissa Hemsley, *The Art of Eating Well* (Ebury
Press, 2014).

28. See the excellent discussion of this in R. Crawford, "Healthism and the
Medicalization of Everyday Life," *International Journal of Health Services* 10,
no. 3 (1980): 365–88.

Chapter 3: How Diet Culture Steals Your Time

1. A. J. Stunkard and M. McLaren-Hume, "The Results of Treatment for
Obesity: A Review of the Literature and Report of a Series," *A.M.A. Archives
of Internal Medicine* 103 (January 1959).

2. Albert Stunkard, "This Week's Citation Classic: Stunkard A. & McLaren-
Hume M. The Results of Treatment for Obesity: A Review of the Literature
and Report of a Series," *Current Contents* 47 (November 21, 1983), http://
garfield.library.upenn.edu/classics1983/A1983RP56700001.pdf.

3. Ottavia Colombo et al., "Is Drop-Out from Obesity Treatment a Predictable
and Preventable Event?," *Nutrition Journal* 13 (February 3, 2014): 13.

4. R. R. Wing and R. W. Jeffrey, "Outpatient Treatment of Obesity: A
Comparison of Methodology and Clinical Results," *International Journal of
Obesity* 3 (1979): 261–79.

5. See, for example, D. Crawford et al., "Can Anyone Successfully Control
Their Weight? Findings of a Three Year Community-Based Study of Men

and Women," *International Journal of Obesity* 24 (2000): 1107–10; A. Fildes et al., "Probability of an Obese Person Attaining Normal Body Weight: Cohort Study Using Electronic Health Records," *American Journal of Public Health* 105 (2015): e54.

6. Jane E. Brody, "Panel Criticizes Weight-Loss Programs," *New York Times,* April 2, 1992, https://www.nytimes.com/1992/04/02/us/panel-criticizes -weight-loss-programs.html.

7. Jane Fritsch, "95% Regain Lost Weight. Or Do They?" *New York Times,* May 25, 1999, https://www.nytimes.com/1999/05/25/health/95-regain-lost -weight-or-do-they.html.

8. Given the 68 percent of Americans who have been on a diet in the past year and the U.S. Census Bureau population estimate of 325,719,178 as of July 1, 2017, there are 221,489,041 dieters.

   When I asked the NWCR media contact for the exact number of people in the registry, he would not cite a more specific number than "more than 10,000." But assuming a generous estimate of 10,999 "successful dieters," that's still only 0.0050 percent (10,999 ÷ 221,489,041 = 0.00004966).

9. J. Ikeda et al., "The National Weight Control Registry: A Critique," *Journal of Nutrition Education and Behavior* 37, no. 4 (July–August 2005): 203–5.

10. Wayne C. Miller, "How Effective Are Traditional Dietary and Exercise Interventions for Weight Loss?," *Medicine & Science in Sports & Exercise* 31, no. 8 (August 1999): 1129–34.

11. Fildes et al., "Probability of an Obese Person Attaining Normal Body Weight," 2015.

12. M. L. Dansinger et al., "Meta-analysis: The Effect of Dietary Counseling for Weight Loss," *Annals of Internal Medicine* 147, no. 1 (2007): 41–50.

13. James W. Anderson et al., "Long-Term Weight-Loss Maintenance: A Meta-analysis of US Studies," *American Journal of Clinical Nutrition* 74 (2001): 579–84.

14. Traci Mann et al., "Medicare's Search for Effective Obesity Treatments: Diets Are Not the Answer," *American Psychologist* 62, no. 3 (April 2007): 220–33.

15. *Ibid.*

16. R. L. Pearl et al., "Weight Bias Internalization and Long-Term Weight Loss in Patients with Obesity," *Annals of Behavioral Medicine,* October 10, 2018.

17. Sandra Aamodt, *Why Diets Make Us Fat* (Current, 2016).

18. C. Logel et al., "Weight Loss Is Not the Answer: A Well-Being Solution to the 'Obesity Problem,'" *Social and Personality Psychology Compass* 9, no. 12 (2015): 678–95.

19. Lindo Bacon, *Health at Every Size: The Surprising Truth About Your Weight,* 2nd edition (BenBella Books, 2010); Aamodt, *Why Diets Make Us Fat,* 2016.

20. C. N. Ochner et al., "Biological Mechanisms That Promote Weight Regain Following Weight Loss in Obese Humans," *Physiology & Behavior* 120 (2013): 106–13.

21. Tara Parker-Pope, "The Fat Trap," *New York Times Magazine,* December 28, 2011.

22. L. M. Gianini, "Long-Term Weight Loss Maintenance in Obesity: Possible Insights from Anorexia Nervosa?," *International Journal of Eating Disorders* 50, no. 4 (2017): 341–42.

23. That's my sweeping overview of a large body of research on health disparities, which is a whole book unto itself. See, for example, L. M. Rivera, "Ethnic-Racial Stigma and Health Disparities: From Psychological Theory and Evidence to Public Policy Solutions," *Journal of Social Issues* 70, no. 2 (2014): 198–205.

24. J. M. Kelso, "Unproven Diagnostic Tests for Adverse Reactions to Foods," *Journal of Allergy and Clinical Immunology: In Practice* 6, no. 2 (2018): 240–50.

25. *Ibid.*

26. *Ibid.*

27. D. L. Beatty Moody et al., "Everyday Discrimination Prospectively Predicts Inflammation Across 7-Years in Racially Diverse Midlife Women: Study of Women's Health Across the Nation," *Journal of Social Issues* 70 (2014): 298–314; Maya Vadiveloo and Josiemer Mattei, "Perceived Weight Discrimination and 10-Year Risk of Allostatic Load Among US Adults," *Annals of Behavioral Medicine* 51, no. 1 (2017): 94–104. (For an in-depth discussion of weight stigma and discrimination, see Chapter 5 of this book, "How Diet Culture Steals Your Well-Being.")

28. A. M. Minihane et al., "Low-Grade Inflammation, Diet Composition and Health: Current Research Evidence and Its Translation," *British Journal of Nutrition* 114, no. 7 (2015): 999–1012; Tufts University Friedman School of Nutrition Science and Policy, "Anti-inflammatory Diets: Do They Work?," *Health & Nutrition Letter,* January 2018, https://www.nutritionletter.tufts.edu/issues/14_1/current-articles/Anti-Inflammatory-Diets-Do-They-Work_2286-1.html.

29. B. Capili et al., "A Clinical Update: Nonceliac Gluten Sensitivity—Is It Really the Gluten?," *Journal for Nurse Practitioners* 10, no. 9 (October 2014): 666–73; J. R. Biesiekierski et al., "Characterization of Adults with a Self-Diagnosis of Nonceliac Gluten Sensitivity," *Nutrition in Clinical Practice* 29, no. 4 (2014): 504–9.

30. J. R. Biesiekierski et al., "No Effects of Gluten in Patients with Self-Reported Non-Celiac Gluten Sensitivity After Dietary Reduction of Fermentable, Poorly Absorbed, Short-Chain Carbohydrates," *Gastroenterology* 145, no. 2 (August 2013): 320–28.

31. Pubmed and Google Scholar searches as of August 30, 2018.

32. H. Herfarth et al., "Prevalence of a Gluten-Free Diet and Improvement of Clinical Symptoms in Patients with Inflammatory Bowel Diseases," *Inflammatory Bowel Diseases* 20, no. 7 (July 2014): 1194–97.

33. P. Hill et al., "Controversies and Recent Developments of the Low-FODMAP Diet," *Gastroenterology & Hepatology* 13, no. 1 (2017): 36; D. Schumann et al., "Randomised Clinical Trial: Yoga vs a Low-FODMAP

Diet in Patients with Irritable Bowel Syndrome," *Alimentary Pharmacology & Therapeutics* 47, no. 2 (2018): 203–11.

34. Hill et al., "Controversies and Recent Developments," 2017.
35. C. Boyd et al., "Psychological Features Are Important Predictors of Functional Gastrointestinal Disorders in Patients with Eating Disorders," *Scandinavian Journal of Gastroenterology* 40, no. 8 (August 2005): 929–35.
36. P. Janssen, "Can Eating Disorders Cause Functional Gastrointestinal Disorders?," *Neurogastroenterology and Motility* 22, no. 12 (December 2010): 1267–69.
37. R. Satherley et al., "Disordered Eating Practices in Gastrointestinal Disorders," *Appetite* 84 (2015): 240–50.
38. A. Mari et al., "Adherence with a Low-FODMAP Diet in Irritable Bowel Syndrome," *European Journal of Gastroenterology & Hepatology* 31, no. 2 (February 2019): 178–82.

Chapter 4: How Diet Culture Steals Your Money

1. Marketdata LLC, "The U.S. Weight Loss and Diet Control Market: A Market Research Analysis," 15th edition (February 2019).
2. South Carolina Department of Mental Health, "Eating Disorder Statistics," 2006, https://www.state.sc.us/dmh/anorexia/statistics.htm, accessed April 4, 2018; L. Reba-Harrelson et al., "Patterns and Prevalence of Disordered Eating and Weight Control Behaviors in Women Ages 25–45," *Eating and Weight Disorders* 14, no. 4 (December 2009): e190–98.
3. J. E. Wildes and M. D. Marcus, "Diagnosis, Assessment, and Treatment Planning for Binge-Eating Disorder and Eating Disorder Not Otherwise Specified," in Carlos M. Grilo and James E. Mitchell, eds., *The Treatment of Eating Disorders: A Clinical Handbook* (New York: Guilford Press, 2010), 45.
4. Coker Capital Advisors, "Monthly Healthcare M&A Update: Sector Spotlight—Eating Disorder Treatment," July 2015, http://cokercapital.com/images/newsletters/2015-July-CCA-Newsletter-Sector-Spotlight-Eating-Disorders-1.pdf, accessed April 17, 2018.
5. C. Jacobi et al., "Coming to Terms with Risk Factors for Eating Disorders: Application of Risk Terminology and Suggestions for a General Taxonomy," *Psychological Bulletin* 130, no. 1 (January 2004): 19–65.
6. S. Hesse-Biber et al., "The Mass Marketing of Disordered Eating and Eating Disorders: The Social Psychology of Women, Thinness and Culture," *Women's Studies International Forum* 29, no. 2 (March–April 2006): 208–24.
7. Virginia Sole-Smith, *The Eating Instinct: Food Culture, Body Image, and Guilt in America* (New York: Henry Holt, 2018).
8. Persistence Market Research, "Global Cold Pressed Juice Market to Reach US $845 Million in Value by 2024-end," February 15, 2017, https://www.persistencemarketresearch.com/mediarelease/cold-pressed-juice-market.asp, accessed April 16, 2018.
9. Shelley Youngblut, "Say You Don't Use Shapewear? Well, Somebody Made Spanx Founder a Billionaire," *Globe and Mail*, March 8, 2012, https://

www.theglobeandmail.com/life/the-hot-button/say-you-dont-use
-shapewear-well-somebody-made-spanx-founder-a-billionaire/
article552273/, accessed April 10, 2018.

10. Erica Schwiegershausen, "Michelle Obama Is a Proud Spanx Wearer,"
The Cut, October 8, 2014, https://www.thecut.com/2014/10/michelle
-obama-is-a-proud-spanx-wearer.html, accessed April 10, 2018.

11. Hiroko Tabuchi, "Spanx Tries to Loosen Up Its Image," *New York Times,*
April 24, 2015, https://www.nytimes.com/2015/04/25/business/spanx
-tries-to-loosen-up-its-image.html, accessed April 10, 2018.

12. Elizabeth Currid-Halkett, "The New, Subtle Ways the Rich Signal Their
Wealth," *BBC Capital,* June 14, 2017, http://www.bbc.com/capital/
story/20170614-the-new-subtle-ways-the-rich-signal-their-wealth?ocid,
accessed April 16, 2018.

13. Molly Langmuir, "What Happens When 'Clean Eating' Turns Into
Obsession?," *Elle,* November 19, 2015, https://www.elle.com/culture/travel
-food/a31411/feeding-frenzy/, accessed April 16, 2018.

14. Abigail C. Saguy, *What's Wrong with Fat?* (Oxford University Press, 2013);
D. Farrell et al., *Accounting for the Cost of US Health Care: A New Look at Why
Americans Spend More,* December 2008, https://www.mckinsey.com/
industries/healthcare-systems-and-services/our-insights/accounting-for
-the-cost-of-us-health-care.

15. Lindo Bacon and Lucy Aphramor, "Weight Science: Evaluating the
Evidence for a Paradigm Shift," *Nutrition Journal* 10, no. 9 (January 2011).

Chapter 5: How Diet Culture Steals Your Well-Being

1. E. Fothergill et al., "Persistent Metabolic Adaptation 6 Years After 'The
Biggest Loser' Competition," *Obesity* 24, no. 8 (August 2016): 1612–19.

2. Rebecca M. Puhl and Chelsea A. Heuer, "Obesity Stigma: Important
Considerations for Public Health," *American Journal of Public Health* 100,
no. 6 (June 2010): 1019–28.

3. E. Han et al., "Weight and Wages: Fat Versus Lean Paychecks," *Health
Economics* 18, no. 5 (May 2009): 535–48.

4. J. M. Hunger et al., "Weighed Down by Stigma: How Weight-Based Social
Identity Threat Contributes to Weight Gain and Poor Health," *Social and
Personality Psychology Compass* 9, no. 6 (June 2015): 255–68.

5. Maya Vadiveloo and Josiemer Mattei, "Perceived Weight Discrimination
and 10-Year Risk of Allostatic Load Among US Adults," *Annals of
Behavioral Medicine* 51, no. 1 (2017): 94–104.

6. M. S. Himmelstein et al., "The Weight of Stigma: Cortisol Reactivity to
Manipulated Weight Stigma," *Obesity* 23, no. 2 (February 2015): 368–74.

7. P. Muennig et al., "I Think Therefore I Am: Perceived Ideal Weight as a
Determinant of Health," *American Journal of Public Health* 98, no. 3 (March
2008): 501–6.

8. A. R. Sutin and A. Terracciano, "Perceived Weight Discrimination and
Obesity," *PLOS ONE* 8, no. 7 (July 2013): e70048.

9. S. E. Jackson and A. Steptoe, "Association Between Perceived Weight Discrimination and Physical Activity: A Population-Based Study Among English Middle-Aged and Older Adults," *BMJ Open* 7, no. 3 (March 2017): e014592.

10. A. J. Tomiyama et al., "How and Why Weight Stigma Drives the Obesity 'Epidemic' and Harms Health," *BMC Medicine* 16, no. 1 (2018): 123.

11. Virgie Tovar, "Take the Cake: The 3 Levels of Fatphobia," *Ravishly,* October 19, 2017, https://ravishly.com/3-levels-of-fatphobia, accessed April 23, 2018.

12. S. M. Phelan et al., "Impact of Weight Bias and Stigma on Quality of Care and Outcomes for Patients with Obesity," *Obesity Reviews* 16, no. 4 (April 2015): 319–26.

13. *Ibid.*

14. Abigail C. Saguy, *What's Wrong with Fat?* (Oxford University Press, 2013).

15. Maya Dusenbery, "Doctors Told Her She Was Just Fat. She Actually Had Cancer," *Cosmopolitan,* April 17, 2018, https://www.cosmopolitan.com/health-fitness/a19608429/medical-fatshaming/.

16. Lindo Bacon and Lucy Aphramor, "Weight Science: Evaluating the Evidence for a Paradigm Shift," *Nutrition Journal* 10, no. 9 (January 2011). Several large-scale studies have shown that people in the so-called "overweight" BMI category actually have the lowest mortality risk of *any* BMI group, while those at the lower end of the "obese" category have about an equal risk with those in the so-called "normal-weight" category. K. M. Flegal et al., "Association of All-Cause Mortality with Overweight and Obesity Using Standard Body Mass Index Categories: A Systematic Review and Meta-analysis," *Jama* 309, no. 1 (January 2, 2013): 71–82.

17. L. Lissner et al., "Variability of Body Weight and Health Outcomes in the Framingham Population," *New England Journal of Medicine* 324 (June 27, 1991): 1839–44.

18. V. A. Diaz et al., "The Association Between Weight Fluctuation and Mortality: Results from a Population-Based Cohort Study," *Journal of Community Health* 30, no. 3 (June 2005): 153–65.

19. M. K. Kim et al., "Associations of Variability in Blood Pressure, Glucose and Cholesterol Concentrations, and Body Mass Index with Mortality and Cardiovascular Outcomes in the General Population," *Circulation* 138, no. 23 (December 4, 2018): 2627–37.

20. J. Montani et al., "Weight Cycling and Cardiometabolic Risks," *Obesity Reviews* 16 (February 2015), Suppl 1: 7–18.

21. M. Schulz et al., "Associations of Short-Term Weight Changes and Weight Cycling with Incidence of Essential Hypertension in the EPIC-Potsdam Study," *Journal of Human Hypertension* 19 (January 2005): 61–67.

22. M. T. Guagnano et al., "Weight Fluctuations Could Increase Blood Pressure in Android Obese Women," *Clinical Sciences* (London) 96, no. 6 (June 1999): 677–80.

23. Montani et al., "Weight Cycling," 2015.

24. Jean Fain, "A Neuroscientist Tackles 'Why Diets Make Us Fat' and Why Mindful Eating Can Help," NPR, June 7, 2016, https://www.npr.org/sections/thesalt/2016/06/07/481094825/a-neuroscientist-tackles-why-diets-make-us-fat.

25. For a discussion of this phenomenon in people with anorexia, see P. E. Rautou et al., "Acute Liver Cell Damage in Patients with Anorexia Nervosa: A Possible Role of Starvation-Induced Hepatocyte Autophagy," *Gastroenterology* 135, no. 3 (September 2008): 840–48.

26. Lindo Bacon, *Health at Every Size: The Surprising Truth About Your Weight,* 2nd edition (BenBella Books, 2010).

27. N. Gletsu-Miller and B. N. Wright, "Mineral Malnutrition Following Bariatric Surgery," *Advances in Nutrition* 4, no. 5 (September 1, 2013): 506–17.

28. J. Tack and E. Deloose, "Complications of Bariatric Surgery: Dumping Syndrome, Reflux and Vitamin Deficiencies," *Best Practice & Research Clinical Gastroenterology* 28, no. 4 (August 2014): 741–49.

29. W. C. King et al., "Prevalence of Alcohol Use Disorders Before and After Bariatric Surgery," *JAMA* 307, no. 23 (June 20, 2012): 2516–25; W. C. King et al., "Alcohol and Other Substance Use After Bariatric Surgery: Prospective Evidence From a U.S. Multicenter Cohort Study," *Surgery for Obesity and Related Diseases* 13, no. 8 (August 2017): 1392–1402.

30. King et al., "Alcohol and Other Substance Use After Bariatric Surgery," 2017.

31. M. L. Westwater et al., "Sugar Addiction: The State of the Science," *European Journal of Nutrition* 55 (November 2016), Suppl 2: 55–69. Also see *Food Psych Podcast,* episode 80, for an in-depth discussion of the clinical problems caused by treating food as an addiction.

32. Linlin Li and Li-Tzy Wu, "Substance Use After Bariatric Surgery: A Review," *Journal of Psychiatric Research* 76 (May 2016): 16–29.

33. D. R. Flum et al., "Early Mortality Among Medicare Beneficiaries Undergoing Bariatric Surgical Procedures," *JAMA* 294, no. 15 (October 19, 2005): 1903–8.

34. The Longitudinal Assessment of Bariatric Surgery (LABS) Consortium et al., "Peri-Operative Safety in the Longitudinal Assessment of Bariatric Surgery," *New England Journal of Medicine* 361, no. 5 (July 30, 2009): 445–54.

35. L. Borish et al., "Death from Anaphylaxis Is a Reassuringly Unusual Outcome," *Journal of Allergy and Clinical Immunology* 133, no. 2 (February 2014): AB234.

36. T. D. Adams et al., "All-Cause and Cause-Specific Mortality Associated with Bariatric Surgery: A Review," *Current Atherosclerosis Reports* 17, no. 12 (December 2015): 74.

37. M. L. Maciejewski et al., "Survival Among High-Risk Patients After Bariatric Surgery," *JAMA* 305, no. 23 (June 15, 2011): 2419–26.

38. D. O. Magro et al., "Long-Term Weight Regain After Gastric Bypass: A 5-Year Prospective Study," *Obesity Surgery* 18, no. 6 (June 2008): 648–51.

39. H. Zheng and C. Chen, "Body Mass Index and Risk of Knee Osteoarthritis: Systematic Review and Meta-analysis of Prospective Studies," *BMJ Open* 5, no. 12 (December 11, 2015): e007568.

Chapter 6: How Diet Culture Steals Your Happiness

1. M. A. Killingsworth and D. T. Gilbert, "A Wandering Mind Is an Unhappy Mind," *Science* 330, no. 6006 (November 12, 2010): 932 LP-932, http://science.sciencemag.org/content/330/6006/932.
2. Sonja Lyubomirsky, *The How of Happiness: A New Approach to Getting the Life You Want* (Penguin Books, 2007).
3. Leah M. Kalm and Richard D. Semba, "They Starved So That Others Be Better Fed: Remembering Ancel Keys and the Minnesota Experiment," *Journal of Nutrition* 135, no. 6 (June 1, 2005): 1347–52.
4. C. Logel et al., "Weight Loss Is Not the Answer: A Well-Being Solution to the 'Obesity Problem,'" *Social and Personality Psychology Compass* 9, no. 12 (2015).
5. See, for example, A. Shcherbina et al., "Accuracy in Wrist-Worn, Sensor-Based Measurements of Heart Rate and Energy Expenditure in a Diverse Cohort," *Journal of Personalized Medicine* 7, no. 2 (2017): 3.
6. E. L. Deci and R. M. Ryan, "Self-Determination Theory: A Macrotheory of Human Motivation, Development, and Health," *Canadian Psychology/ Psychologie Canadienne* 49, no. 3 (2008): 182–85.
7. Bob Greene, "Oprah's Weight Loss Confession," oprah.com, January 5, 2009, https://www.oprah.com/health/oprahs-weight-loss-confession.
8. S. Täuber, "Moralized Health-Related Persuasion Undermines Social Cohesion," *Frontiers in Psychology* 9 (2018): 909.
9. C. Evers et al., "Feeling Bad or Feeling Good, Does Emotion Affect Your Consumption of Food? A Meta-analysis of the Experimental Evidence," *Neuroscience & Biobehavioral Reviews* 92 (September 2018): 195–208.
10. T. L. Tylka et al., "Is Intuitive Eating the Same as Flexible Dietary Control? Their Links to Each Other and Well-Being Could Provide an Answer," *Appetite* 95 (December 2015): 166–75; J. Linardon and S. Mitchell, "Rigid Dietary Control, Flexible Dietary Control, and Intuitive Eating: Evidence for Their Differential Relationship to Disordered Eating and Body Image Concerns," *Eating Behaviors* 26 (August 2017): 16–22.
11. P. Bongers and A. Jansen, "Emotional Eating Is Not What You Think It Is and Emotional Eating Scales Do Not Measure What You Think They Measure," *Frontiers in Psychology* 7 (2016): 1932.

Chapter 7: Enough Is Enough

1. Laurie Penny, "Most Women You Know Are Angry—and That's All Right," *Teen Vogue*, August 2, 2017, https://www.teenvogue.com/story/women-angry-anger-laurie-penny, accessed July 3, 2018.
2. Leslie Jamison, "I Used to Insist I Didn't Get Angry. Not Anymore," *New York Times Magazine*, January 17, 2018, https://www.nytimes.com/2018/01/17/magazine/i-used-to-insist-i-didnt-get-angry-not-anymore.html, accessed July 3, 2018.

3. A. C. Kelly and G. A. Tasca, "Within-Persons Predictors of Change During Eating Disorders Treatment: An Examination of Self-Compassion, Self-Criticism, Shame, and Eating Disorder Symptoms," *International Journal of Eating Disorders* 49, no. 7 (2016): 716–22, http://doi.org/10.1002/eat .22527.

4. Kristin Neff, *Self-Compassion: The Proven Power of Being Kind to Yourself* (William Morrow, 2011).

5. See E. R. Albertson et al., "Self-Compassion and Body Dissatisfaction in Women: A Randomized Controlled Trial of a Brief Meditation Intervention," *Mindfulness* 6, no. 3 (2015): 444–54; C. Ferreira et al., "Self-Compassion in the Face of Shame and Body Image Dissatisfaction: Implications for Eating Disorders," *Eating Behaviors* 14, no. 2 (2013): 207–10.

6. T. L. Tylka et al., "Is Intuitive Eating the Same as Flexible Dietary Control? Their Links to Each Other and Well-Being Could Provide an Answer," *Appetite* 95 (December 2015).

Chapter 8: Reclaim Your Right to Eat Intuitively

1. Evelyn Tribole and Elyse Resch, *Intuitive Eating: A Revolutionary Program That Works* (St. Martin's Griffin, 2012).

2. *Ibid.*

3. J. Polivy and C. P. Herman, "Restrained Eating and Food Cues: Recent Findings and Conclusions," *Current Obesity Reports* 6, no. 1 (2017): 79–85.

4. Anahad O'Connor, "More Evidence That Nutrition Studies Don't Always Add Up," *New York Times*, September 29, 2018, https://www.nytimes .com/2018/09/29/sunday-review/cornell-food-scientist-wansink -misconduct.html.

5. A. J. Tomiyama et al., "Low Calorie Dieting Increases Cortisol," *Psychosomatic Medicine* 72, no. 4 (May 2010): 357–64.

6. Leah M. Kalm and Richard D. Semba, "They Starved So That Others Be Better Fed: Remembering Ancel Keys and the Minnesota Experiment," *Journal of Nutrition* 135, no. 6 (June 1, 2005).

7. C. B. Becker et al., "Food Insecurity and Eating Disorder Pathology," *International Journal of Eating Disorders* 50, no. 9 (September 2017): 1031–40.

Chapter 9: Stop Labeling Food as **Good** *or* **Bad**

1. Maya Vadiveloo and Josiemer Mattei, "Perceived Weight Discrimination and 10-Year Risk of Allostatic Load Among US Adults," *Annals of Behavioral Medicine* 51, no. 1 (2017): 94–104.

2. T. L. Tylka et al., "Is Intuitive Eating the Same as Flexible Dietary Control? Their Links to Each Other and Well-Being Could Provide an Answer," *Appetite* 95 (December 2015).

3. J. Polivy et al., "The Effect of Deprivation on Food Cravings and Eating Behavior in Restrained and Unrestrained Eaters," *International Journal of Eating Disorders* 38, no. 4 (2005): 301–9.

4. T. Smith and S. R. Hawks, "Intuitive Eating, Diet Composition, and the Meaning of Food in Healthy Weight Promotion," *American Journal of Health Education* 37, no. 3 (2006): 130–36.

5. *Ibid.*; G. Hawley et al., "Sustainability of Health and Lifestyle Improvements Following a Non-dieting Randomised Trial in Overweight Women," *Preventive Medicine* 47, no. 6 (December 2008): 593–99.

6. Smith and Hawks, "Intuitive Eating," 2006; C. E. Madden et al., "Eating in Response to Hunger and Satiety Signals Is Related to BMI in a Nationwide Sample of 1601 Mid-age New Zealand Women," *Public Health Nutrition* 15, no. 12 (December 2012): 2272–79.

7. C. Bennette and A. Vickers, "Against Quantiles: Categorization of Continuous Variables in Epidemiologic Research, and Its Discontents," *BMC Medical Research Methodology* 12, no. 21 (February 29, 2012).

8. K. L. Stanhope, "Sugar Consumption, Metabolic Disease and Obesity: The State of the Controversy," *Critical Reviews in Clinical Laboratory Sciences* 53, no. 1 (2016): 52–67.

9. See Q. Yang et al., "Added Sugar Intake and Cardiovascular Diseases Mortality Among US Adults," *JAMA Internal Medicine* 174, no. 4 (April 2014): 516–24. In this book I've deliberately omitted mentioning the numeric percentage of calories from sugar because I want to avoid triggering diet-culture thinking in readers' minds. My calculations of food equivalents, however, are based on the numeric values described in the above study, plus manufacturer-reported nutrition facts.

10. Abigail C. Saguy, *What's Wrong with Fat?* (Oxford University Press, 2013).

11. A. Sutin et al., "Weight Discrimination and Unhealthy Eating-Related Behaviors," *Appetite* 102 (2016): 83–89; A. J. Tomiyama and T. Mann, "If Shaming Reduced Obesity, There Would Be No Fat People," *Hastings Center Report* 43, no. 3 (2013): 4–5.

12. M. R. Sardar et al., "Cardiovascular Impact of Eating Disorders in Adults: A Single Center Experience and Literature Review," *Heart Views: The Official Journal of the Gulf Heart Association* 16, no. 3 (July–September 2015): 88–92; V. A. Diaz et al., "The Association Between Weight Fluctuation and Mortality Results from a Population-Based Cohort Study," *Journal of Community Health* 30, no. 3 (June 2005): 153–65; Maya Vadiveloo and Josiemer Mattei, "Perceived Weight Discrimination and 10-Year Risk of Allostatic Load Among US Adults," *Annals of Behavioral Medicine* 51, no. 1 (2017): 94–104.

13. M. L. Westwater et al., "Sugar Addiction: The State of the Science," *European Journal of Nutrition* 55 (November 2016), Suppl 2: 55–69.

14. L. H. Sweet et al., "Brain Response to Food Stimulation in Obese, Normal Weight, and Successful Weight Loss Maintainers," *Obesity* 20, no. 11 (November 2012): 2220–25.

15. Saguy, *What's Wrong with Fat?*, 2013.

16. H. Park et al., "Relative Contributions of a Set of Health Factors to Selected Health Outcomes," *American Journal of Preventive Medicine* 49, no. 6 (2015): 961–69; C. Hood et al., "County Health Rankings: Relationships

Between Determinant Factors and Health Outcomes," *American Journal of Preventive Medicine* 50, no. 2 (February 2016): 129–35.

17. Saguy, *What's Wrong with Fat?*, 2013.

18. R. M. Puhl and K. D. Brownell, "Confronting and Coping with Weight Stigma: An Investigation of Overweight and Obese Adults," *Obesity* 14, no. 10 (2006): 1802–15.

19. J. A. Sabin et al., "Implicit and Explicit Anti-Fat Bias Among a Large Sample of Medical Doctors by BMI, Race/Ethnicity and Gender," *PLOS ONE* 7, no. 11 (November 7, 2012): e48448.

20. K. Tremelling et al., "Orthorexia Nervosa and Eating Disorder Symptoms in Registered Dietitian Nutritionists in the United States," *Journal of the Academy of Nutrition and Dietetics* 117, no. 10 (October 2017): 1612–17.

Chapter 10: Health at Every Size—and Body Liberation

1. Association for Size Diversity and Health, "HAES® Principles" (no date), https://www.sizediversityandhealth.org/content.asp?id=152, accessed August 17, 2018.

2. A. J. Tomiyama et al., "Misclassification of Cardiometabolic Health When Using Body Mass Index Categories in NHANES 2005–2012," *International Journal of Obesity* 40, no. 5 (2016): 883–86.

3. That includes conferences put on by the Academy for Eating Disorders (AED), the National Eating Disorders Association (NEDA), the International Association of Eating Disorder Professionals (IAEDP), the Binge Eating Disorder Association (BEDA), the Renfrew Center Foundation, and the Multi-Service Eating Disorders Association (MEDA).

4. Lindo Bacon and Lucy Aphramor, *Body Respect: What Conventional Health Books Get Wrong, Leave Out, and Just Plain Fail to Understand About Weight* (BenBella Books, 2014).

5. Be Nourished, "What Is Body Trust®?" (no date), https://benourished
.org/about-body-trust/, accessed August 22, 2018.

Chapter 11: The Power of Community

1. P. Muennig et al., "I Think Therefore I Am: Perceived Ideal Weight as a Determinant of Health," *American Journal of Public Health* 98, no. 3 (March 2008): 501–6.

2. J. W. Dearing, "Applying Diffusion of Innovation Theory to Intervention Development," *Research on Social Work Practice* 19, no. 5 (September 1, 2009): 503–18.

Index

Questions and Topics for Discussion

> *Diet culture*—a system of beliefs that equates thinness, muscularity, and particular body shapes with health and moral virtue; promotes weight loss and body reshaping as a means of attaining higher status; demonizes certain foods and food groups while elevating others; and oppresses people who don't match its supposed picture of "health."
>
> — CHRISTY HARRISON, *Anti-Diet*

1. What are some examples of toxic diet culture that you are confronted with in your day-to-day life?

2. Throughout history, there have been endless diet trends and weight-loss programs. How have these changed over time? How have they stayed the same?

3. Diet culture and body shaming are pervasive in the media. What are some recent news stories that you have identified as problematic after reading *Anti-Diet*?

4. Christy Harrison calls out the sexist, racist, classist, and ableist nature of diet culture. What are some examples from the book that you found especially illuminating? Have you experienced them in your own life?

5. In 2019 Marketdata reported that the U.S. diet industry is worth more than $72 billion. What are some ways in which you have contributed money to the diet industry in the past that you may have been unaware of before reading this book?

6. Today we see a shift toward "wellness" trends. Why are these still problematic to our health?

7. How is intuitive eating different from dieting?

8. Have you made any changes to your eating and movement practices after reading *Anti-Diet*? Are there any "anti-diet" communities where you live? If not, what are some first steps one could take to create such a community?

About the Author

Christy Harrison, MPH, RD, is a registered dietitian nutritionist, certified intuitive eating counselor, and journalist who has been covering food and nutrition for more than sixteen years. Through her private practice and popular podcast, *Food Psych,* she's helped tens of thousands of people around the world stop dieting, recover from disordered eating, and make peace with food and their bodies. She speaks regularly at professional conferences, colleges, and webinars to train fellow clinicians on intuitive eating and the anti-diet approach. Find her at christyharrison.com and @chr1styharrison.